FIND YOUR FIT

FIND YOUR FIT

A Nurse's Guide to Choosing
the Right Unit

By Dayna Vidal, DNP, RN
The Recovering Nurse Executive™

Find Your Fit: A Nurse's Guide to Choosing the Right Unit

Copyright ©2025 Simply Stellar Nursing

All rights reserved. No portion of this book may be reproduced in any form, by any means, electronic or mechanical, including photocopying, recording, or by any information storage and retrieval system, without permission in writing from the publisher.

987654321
First Edition
Printed in the United States of America.

Cover design by Jake Clark, Pithy Wordsmithery
Interior layout by Sue Murray, Pithy Wordsmithery
Copyediting by Nils Kuehn, Pithy Wordsmithery
Proofreading by Scott Morrow and Katharine Dvorak, Pithy Wordsmithery

ISBN: 979-8-9997978-5-8 (paperback)
ISBN: 979-8-9997978-7-2 (e-book)
ISBN: 979-8-9997978-6-5 (hardcover)

Dayna Vidal, DNP, RN
Email: dr.day@therecoveringnurseexecutive.com
Website: therecoveringnurseexecutive.com

Library of Congress Control Number: 2025917313

Endorsements

"*Find Your Fit* is the book nurses didn't know they desperately needed. With compassion and clarity, Dr. Dayna Vidal puts words to a struggle that many experience but few know how to articulate—feeling misplaced in the very profession they love. Her storytelling is emotionally honest, clinically grounded, and refreshingly actionable. I've worked closely with new nurses who doubted their abilities simply because they were in the wrong environment. This book offers insight and tools to change that trajectory. It's a timely, transformative guide that will help nurses not just stay in the profession but thrive in it."

—Alice Benjamin, Media Strategist, MediaRX

"*Find Your Fit* is the book I wish every new nurse—and every nurse leader—had on their shelf. Dr. Dayna Vidal delivers an honest, insightful, and research-backed guide that reframes how we think about nurse retention, burnout, and professional fulfillment. Through compelling stories and clear, actionable chapters, she shows that it's not about whether someone is 'cut out' for nursing—it's about helping them find the right environment to thrive.

Dayna brings the heart of a nurse and the mind of a strategist, and her message is both urgent and empowering: nurses don't leave the profession because they lack passion—they often leave because they were placed in a setting misaligned with their strengths. This book helps nurses make informed, self-aware decisions about their careers, and it equips leaders to foster better support systems from the start.

Whether you're a nursing student, a newly licensed RN, or a seasoned clinician reconsidering your next move, *Find Your Fit* is an essential road map for building a sustainable and joyful nursing career. I wholeheartedly recommend it."

—Dr. Bob Dent, DNP, MBA, RN, NEA-BC, ACC, FACHE, FAAN, FAONL
Past President, American Organization for Nursing Leadership
Co-Author of the James A. Hamilton Award–Winning Book, *Building a Culture of Ownership in Healthcare*

"Dayna has written the book every nurse wishes they had at the start of their career—and the one many seasoned nurses didn't realize they needed. With deep insight and genuine compassion, *Find Your Fit* addresses one of the most overlooked factors in burnout: misalignment between a nurse's strengths and their environment. Dayna's guidance helps readers make sense of their experiences and empowers them to make informed, confident decisions about where and how they practice. I hired Dayna as a new graduate and have had the privilege of watching her evolve into a remarkable leader, educator, and advocate for nurses. Her voice is both timely and timeless."

—Elaina McAdams, DNP, RN, MBA, NEA-BC, FACHE
Founder/CEO, CAUHEC Connect

"Dr. Vidal has brought a significant topic to the reader that is missing from the shelves and touched on the biggest factor in a new nurse's success: finding the right fit. As an experienced executive and a leader who is seeking the most optimal plan for onboarding and retention, I cannot wait to share this content with my team and new nurses entering the profession. I look forward to using this book as a model for onboarding our student nurse externs and interns. We have been trying to write about the personas of what nursing looks like in each of our departments. These stories and Dr. Vidal's guidance bring those personas to life in a way that will foster confidence and support our future nursing generations."

—Kim Reddish, PhD, RN, CCRN, CENP, Chief Nurse Executive,
Forrest Health System

Dedication

For my family.

To my mother and father, your sacrifices built the foundation I stand on. You taught me to value wisdom over status, courage over comfort, and love over everything. Every part of this book carries your legacy.

To my sister, thank you for being my mirror, my anchor, and my lifelong reminder that I am never walking alone.

To my son and daughter, your presence is my purpose. You are the clearest evidence that love can be both fierce and gentle. Watching you become who you are reminds me daily why this work must be done with integrity.

To my husband, thank you for being my sanctuary. For holding space when the world felt too heavy. For never asking me to shrink. Your steady support made this possible.

And to the nurses...

The ones who have been.
The ones who are still becoming.
The ones who feel like they're breaking.
The ones who keep showing up anyway.

This is for you.
Your story matters.
Your voice is valid.
You deserve a career that sees your whole humanity.

Table of Contents

Foreword — xi
Preface — xv
Introduction — xxi

CHAPTER 1: Unit Vibes — 1

CHAPTER 2: Personality Self-Assessment — 17

CHAPTER 3: Consider the Pace — 25

CHAPTER 4: Emotional Investment — 35

CHAPTER 5: Work-Life Balance — 43

CHAPTER 6: You've Got the Power — 53

CHAPTER 7: Tech It or Leave It — 63

CHAPTER 8: Variety — 71

CHAPTER 9: Like You, Every Hospital Has Its Own Personality — 79

CHAPTER 10: Gut Check — 91

CHAPTER 11: Go All In — 99

CHAPTER 12: Your Journey from Self-Doubt to Self-Confidence — 109

Acknowledgments — 121
About the Author — 125

Foreword

When Dr. Vidal shared *Find Your Fit: A Nurse's Guide to Choosing the Right Unit* with me, I knew she was tackling something we don't talk about nearly enough in nursing: just how much your work environment can make or break your career. This isn't another "how to get a nursing job" book. It's about setting yourself up to actually succeed and love what you do. My own research and scholarship have centered on how nurses develop clinical expertise over time, particularly through experiential learning in real-world settings. The *From Novice to Expert* model, grounded in the Dreyfus Model of Skill Acquisition, identifies five stages of development in nursing practice: novice, advanced beginner, competent, proficient, and expert. This model emphasizes that clinical knowledge is not static or simply academic. *Find Your Fit* is shaped and deepened through context, practice, and reflection. The capacity to notice significant changes, respond intuitively to patient needs, and engage ethically and compassionately emerges over time in environments that support growth.

That's exactly what Dr. Vidal gets at in this book. She's seen it happen over and over: a bright, capable nurse who's totally committed to the profession ends up struggling and thinking maybe nursing isn't for her. But often, it's not about the nurse at all. It's about the mismatch between who they are and where they're working. Without the right environmental conditions, even the most dedicated nurses can get stuck at earlier stages of development, never fully realizing their potential.

What I love about *Find Your Fit* is how practical it is. Dr. Vidal gives readers a map. She combines personal stories from real nurses, vivid clinical scenarios, and actionable strategies to help nurses identify what environments actually support their strengths. She doesn't shy away from the complexity or emotional labor of this work, but she also doesn't leave nurses stuck in the overwhelm. She walks them through it, chapter by chapter. Rather than just telling you that environment matters, she gives you concrete ways to figure out what kind of environment will work for you, connecting your personality, strengths, and what energizes versus drains you to the reality of different units. Honestly, working in the ER requires a completely different mindset than working in hospice or pediatrics.

You can tell that this book comes from someone who's been in the trenches. Dr. Vidal writes with the kind of clarity that comes from watching countless nurses either flourish or burn out and understanding that the difference often comes down to finding the right fit. For anyone involved in training or supporting new nurses, whether you're an educator, a preceptor, or running a residency program, this book offers frameworks you can actually use to help people make better choices about where they start their careers.

But this matters beyond just individual nurses. With burnout rates through the roof and people leaving the profession faster than we can replace them, Dr. Vidal is pointing toward something that health systems really need to hear. Yes, better pay and schedules matter, but so does making sure people are working in places where they can actually use their strengths and grow into the nurses that we desperately need them to become.

What I appreciate most is that this book doesn't try to fit everyone into the same mold. It recognizes that both nurses and nursing units are incredibly diverse, and that's actually a good thing. Instead of prescribing one right way to do things, it encourages honest self-reflection and real conversations about what success looks like for each person.

Foreword

I'm recommending this book to nursing students who are trying to figure out where to start, to new grads who might be second-guessing their choices, and especially to the educators and managers who are trying to support them. Even experienced nurses thinking about making a change will find value here. It's a reminder that where you work matters just as much as how hard you work, and finding that right fit can be the difference between loving your career and walking away from it entirely.

—**Dr. Patricia Benner, RN, PhD, FAAN**

Preface

It doesn't feel like that long ago when I was a nurse extern in a burn unit, a nursing student with no real idea about the journey I was starting or how it was going to transform me into the person I see in the mirror today. That journey took me from that burn unit to the boardroom as a nurse executive. My career unfolded in ways that felt both inevitable and improbable. It was a path I never planned but one that, looking back, feels as if it had been waiting for me all along.

Though I've learned many life lessons along the way, one of the most important ones came during my most recent leadership role. As a nursing leader, I realized that supporting nurses both as they enter and as they progress in this rewarding profession requires more than just guidance. It demands intentional support and strategic placement in helping them find the right fit.

It was a few years ago when I became vice president of nursing professional development, education, and quality, responsible for the nurse residency program. I was determined to be more than just a distant figure in the hospital hierarchy. I needed to understand the reality of the nurses who I was supposed to support—the ones fresh out of school, bravely choosing to help patients despite the chaos of the COVID-19 pandemic, clinging to the idealism that had carried them through endless nights of studying and clinical rotations. If I were going to make a difference, I had to be in the trenches with them, making their struggles my own.

It was during those first couple of months when I met Kelli. She was still a nursing student then, anxiously preparing for the

NCLEX (National Council Licensure Examination), that final gatekeeper standing between her and the career that she had spent years working toward. She was bright, eager, and full of an unshakeable confidence that made you believe she would thrive in any unit that would be fortunate enough to get her. But she wanted the emergency department and only the emergency department.

I gave her my email, and she reached out to me a few times for tips and reassurance that the NCLEX wasn't as intimidating as everyone made it seem. I gave her all the information I could, including some words of encouragement here and there. Ultimately, as I knew she would, Kelli passed the NCLEX and landed a position in her dream ED unit.

And that, I thought, was the beginning of a great nursing career.

I saw Kelli often during her first couple of months as she progressed through orientation, and she seemed to be doing well. Fast-forward six months when Kelli was taking full patient assignments and settling into her new life as a professional registered nurse.

I noticed her sitting alone in one of the nursing classrooms, scrolling through her phone while waiting for her monthly residency meeting to begin.

"Kelli?" I inquired.

She looked up, startled, and then broke into a smile and jumped up to hug me.

It wasn't until I pulled back that I saw her—I mean REALLY saw her.

Gone was the confident, energetic young woman I had met months earlier. She had lost at least 15 pounds off her already thin frame, and the exhaustion was etched into the dark circles underneath her hollowed eyes. The spark that had once made her shine had been replaced with something duller, something defeated.

Preface

"Let's go to my office," I offered.

As soon as the door to my office was closed, silent tears began rolling down her cheeks, and just like those tears, it didn't take long for her story to spill out.

"Well, it happened like two weeks ago," she began.

With a dazed look, as if she were suddenly in another time and place, Kelli's words filled my office as she described the scene in a way that made me feel in the middle of it all:

> I tighten the straps on my N95 and adjust my face shield, smudged with sweat and God knows what else. My ears ache from hours of pressure thanks to the elastic straps stretching across the back of my head, but there's no time to care about that now. The ER is a war zone tonight.
>
> The first code came in right at the beginning of my shift: a guy about my age, found unresponsive at a music festival. Overdose. We barely got the tube in before his stats tanked. Now he's sedated, intubated, and likely to become another statistic.
>
> Fifteen minutes later, another OD rolls in. Young mom. Paramedics said they found her slumped on the couch while her two-year-old wandered the apartment alone. My stomach twists, but I shove it down. No time to feel...that will have to come later.
>
> By 20:00, I've lost track of how many rapid responses I've run to. I'm pushing a bed into the elevator when a voice cuts through the chaos.
>
> "Kelli, we need you now! Another one's crashing."
>
> I sprint, sneakers sticking to the floor—hopefully sweat, maybe coffee, more than likely something worse.
>
> Room 41. Elderly man. COVID pneumonia. He's drowning in his own lungs, eyes wide open, and terrified as he gasps for air. The monitor flashes "64% SpO_2."
>
> "Start bagging him!" my preceptor shouts over the commotion.
>
> The doctor calls for RSI. I draw up etomidate, then succinylcholine, my hands moving on autopilot. The resident fumbles with the laryngoscope.

> *"I can't see the cords!" he shouts.*
>
> *I reach up and adjust the bright exam light, momentarily blinding myself.*
>
> *Another attempt. A brutal, tense few seconds. Then, finally, the tube slides in. A respiratory therapist secures it. I step back, head swimming.*
>
> *I realize, suddenly, that I haven't taken a real breath in hours. My left eyelid starts to twitch, and the dull headache I had all morning starts to become a full migraine.*
>
> *"Kelli, can you..."*
>
> *"I just need a second."*
>
> *Without waiting for permission, I push past a tech, past the alarms and beeping monitors, past the chaos, and head for the supply room.*
>
> *I yank the door shut behind me. Clean. Quiet. Safe.*
>
> *My chest feels tight, and I try to take in deep breaths. "It's fine," I tell myself. "I'm OK. This is how it is every day...just another shift."*
>
> *Except I'm not OK.*
>
> *Because when I blink, I'm back in room 41, watching the patient's hands grasp at nothing, seeing the festival kid seize on the stretcher, remembering the sight of the young mom's lips turning blue.*
>
> *My hands won't stop shaking.*
>
> *I slide down to the floor, arms wrapped around my knees. I should get up. I should walk back out there like I always do.*
>
> *But for the first time, I'm afraid that if I do, I'll never find my way back to myself.*
>
> *And that scares me more than any code ever could.*

My heart went out to her. It was easy to see that Kelli's experience in the ED had shaken her confidence and shattered her idealistic view of the nursing profession. She had realized the cost of her dream and wondered whether she could still afford to pay it. What frustrated her most was that the other new nurses were thriving, showing up to the ED every day filled with excitement

Preface

and energy. Sure, they were exhausted by the end of their shifts despite the energy drinks and cups of coffee, but they were fulfilled, satisfied. She truly believed that she had made a mistake by choosing the ED and, more importantly, choosing to be a nurse.

I was devastated for Kelli, but more than that, I was disappointed in myself as an experienced nurse leader and professional development "expert" responsible for helping nurses like her. Patient-care leaders usually go into interviews to determine whether a candidate is a good fit for their unit. *We've been approaching this all wrong*, I thought to myself. It's not that Kelli wasn't a good fit for nursing or for the ED. The ED was not a good fit for her!

This was my lightbulb moment.

Over the years, I saw countless nurses struggle and even leave the profession entirely, not because they didn't want to care for others but because they were simply in the wrong unit, a unit that did not align with their strengths and skills. As I looked back, I realized that this profession has lost far too many compassionate, talented, skilled nurses who had concluded that nursing wasn't for them anymore because they were burned out. But what they didn't understand was the reason they were burned out: it wasn't about being a nurse; it was about working in the wrong environment.

Yes, we need to remember why we chose nursing overall and remember our passion for this career, but we also need to understand that there are different environments, different units that require different skills and capabilities. This point is equally as important as remembering our passion to care for others. Yet no one is talking about it.

That's exactly why I decided to write this book!

Introduction

The nursing profession is filled with all kinds of stories. Some end beautifully, with nurses feeling so fulfilled that they cannot imagine a life that didn't include caring for others day in and day out. They thrive until the day they decide to retire. Other stories end in turmoil, with nurses feeling unfulfilled, burned out, and miserable. They walk out in search of another profession, wondering how they got so off course.

Take, for example, Gabriella, a fresh-faced, eager nurse, ready to make a difference. The day she first stepped onto the floor, she couldn't wait to dive into patient care, connecting with patients and offering comfort and support. But when she was placed in a unit where the pace was relentless and the tasks felt disconnected from her passion, her excitement quickly turned to dread. Every shift felt like a battle. And soon, Gabriella found herself counting the minutes until she could leave, wondering if nursing was truly the right path for her. This wasn't what she had imagined at all! Frustrated and exhausted, she made the heart-wrenching decision to walk away, convinced that she had chosen the wrong profession.

But was it really the profession? Or was it simply the wrong fit?
These are the questions this book explores.

Whether you've been rocking your scrubs for 3 days or 30 years, I want you to start by taking a moment to hype yourself up. You've stepped into a career that's more than just a job. Nursing is a source of pride, an outlet for passion, and a foundation for purpose. In fact, nursing has been voted the most trusted profession for the past 23 years in a row.[i] Before we dive into the details about finding the right fit, pause, take a breath, and give yourself some credit—you've earned it!

But let's also be real. Though nursing is incredibly rewarding, it's undeniably tough. Everyone will tell you how fulfilling it can be, and they're not wrong. But that doesn't make it any easier. Even in the perfect hospital, with the best team, in a unit that feels like home, nursing is still demanding. Now imagine you're in a hospital that's far from perfect (spoiler: none of them are perfect) or working with an amazing but very human team (translation: nobody's perfect). Then imagine that you are in a department that just doesn't align with your strengths or personality. Under such conditions, even the best nurses would struggle.

That's when burnout creeps in, making you question whether you belong in nursing at all. For new nurses, it's particularly important to prevent burnout, as about **1 in 3 leave** within their first **two to three years** because of burnout, often stemming from not finding the right fit.[ii] Instead of being energized every day, full of passion, they feel depleted and exhausted.

Like most nurses, you might be wondering how you should manage your time, worrying about making mistakes that could harm patients, or struggling with work-life balance and the overwhelming workload. I've been there. And after over 15 years in nursing (including several years in executive leadership and professional development), I've seen countless nurses navigate these same challenges while wasting years trying to figure out where they belong. Many bounce from unit to unit, or even from hospital to hospital, searching for where they belong. And though there's nothing wrong with exploring different areas, it's heartbreaking when great nurses burn out or leave the profession entirely, thinking that they're just not cut out for it.

That's exactly why I wrote this book for experienced nurses considering a change, nursing students, and new nurses alike. *Find Your Fit* is here to help you discover a nursing unit where you feel like you belong. No matter where we each are in our

Introduction

careers, we all share the same concerns. My hope is that this book eases those worries so you can create the career you've always wanted and become the nurse you've dreamed of being.

It's about understanding that every department has its own unique set of demands, from the fast-paced, high-stress environment of the ER to the more methodical, detail-oriented work in a clinical setting. Each department requires specific skills, the right mindset, and clinical expertise, whether it's the ability to make quick decisions under pressure in the ICU or the patience and communication skills necessary in palliative care. Understanding these nuances will empower you not only to navigate the diverse roles in nursing but also to find the one that truly aligns with your strengths.

Choosing the right unit "vibe" is incredibly important for long-term job satisfaction and career longevity. When you align with a unit that matches your personality and work style, you're more likely to experience fulfillment and growth.[iii] The right vibe not only makes day-to-day tasks easier and more enjoyable, but it also improves emotional resilience, helping you handle the inevitable challenges that nursing brings with a positive outlook. Working in an environment that feels right for you provides the space for both personal growth and professional development, ultimately leading to a more rewarding nursing career.

Throughout the following pages, you'll find real experiences, insights, and resources to help you avoid unnecessary struggles and charge into your role with confidence. How exactly do we move from the "Island of Anxiety" to the "Land of Confidence"? We are going to take this journey together in the following three steps:

1. Review the inner workings of the most common departments in the hospital (chapter 1).
2. Discuss how to objectively take inventory of your personality (chapter 2).

3. Explore how certain personality traits align with success on various units (chapters 3–8).

After that, I share tips I've learned over the years as a nursing professional development leader on how to successfully start your nursing career or pivot into a new specialty. I also touch on career pathways and take a sneak peek at ways to adapt and reevaluate your journey as you grow professionally and transform personally over time.

The goal of this book is simple: to help you figure out where *you* fit. What unit aligns with your personality, your skills, and your long-term goals? *Find Your Fit* is here to help you discover where your natural talents and skills best align with the needs of various departments. Whether you're a seasoned nurse or just starting your career, aligning your strengths with the right role in the right unit can lead to a nursing journey that is personally fulfilling and financially freeing.

Do you ever feel like everyone else on the unit or in your clinical rotation group just *knows what they're doing*—and you're the only one second-guessing every move you make? That's not failure. That's *development* supported by actual research.

That's Patricia Benner's *From Novice to Expert* theory playing out in real time.[iv]

Benner wasn't just talking about clinical skill levels. She was naming what so many of us felt but didn't have words for: how a nurse grows through experience. How we move from rule-following novices to intuitive experts. And most importantly? How that growth doesn't happen in a vacuum.

It happens in context.

It happens in culture.

It happens when a nurse is placed in the right environment to *learn*, *belong*, and *bloom*.

As you dive into this book, you'll gain insights into how to assess different nursing specialties, identify where your skills

Introduction

shine the brightest, and position yourself for long-term success. Get ready to explore how you can maximize your potential and thrive in this dynamic field because finding your fit is about unlocking your full potential and finding true fulfillment in your nursing career. There's no time like the present.

In the first chapter, we look at some of the most common units in the hospital in terms of their "vibe," so grab your stethoscope, slip on your scrubs, and let's get started!

CHAPTER 1

Unit Vibes

Welcome to the ultimate vibe check! Choosing the right nursing unit goes way beyond filling out an application. It's about finding your work home away from home. Whether you're craving the fast-paced action of the ER or the deep human connections in oncology, every unit has its own rhythm and energy.

That's what we are talking about here. When I say "unit vibe," I am talking about the collective atmosphere, culture, and energy of a nursing unit. It's the emotional tone and work dynamic that influences how the team communicates, works together, and supports one another. Some of the people you work with will feel like family members. You will work shoulder to shoulder and likely spend more waking hours with them than with your friends and family outside the hospital, so it's important that you share some commonalities and like each other. Simply, those you work with are a big part of the unit vibe. Whether the unit is fast-paced and adrenaline-driven, like the ER, or compassionate and relationship-based, like oncology, the vibe of a unit shapes daily interactions and impacts the overall work experience.

In this chapter, we're diving into what makes each nursing unit unique so you can find the perfect match for

Broken bones, sick hearts, disturbed minds: people come to the hospital for all kinds of reasons, and the nursing units that care for them are just as different. Each unit has its own energy, pace, and personality. Finding the one that best fits you is the secret to loving what you do.

your personality, work style, and career goals. Ready to vibe with your future nursing squad?

Types of Nursing Units and Their Vibes

Broken bones, sick hearts, disturbed minds: people come to the hospital for all kinds of reasons, and the nursing units that care for them are just as different. Each unit has its own energy, pace, and personality. Finding the one that best fits you is the secret to loving what you do.

Emergency Department

Working in the emergency room feels like stepping into a world of controlled chaos. Here, predictability goes out the window and every second can change the rhythm of your entire shift. There is an energy in the ER, where everyone is hustling to make sure things stay on track. To outsiders, it might seem like pure pandemonium, but for the team of clinicians and support staff who work there, it's a beautiful commotion with a purpose.

Congested hallways are packed with stretchers, carts, and all sorts of equipment, with everyone finding ways to slip past each other as they rush to wherever they're needed the most. You better believe that everyone knows their role, whether it's stabilizing a patient, prepping a room, or hunting down needed supplies. It's like a turbulent dance where every step is rehearsed and every person understands their part.

The ER is also a crossroads, where people from every background and socioeconomic level seek care—everyone has their own story to tell, a story as unique as their fingerprints and DNA. One minute, you're treating a homeless person suffering from long-neglected health issues, and the next, you're caring for a business executive who's just been in a devastating car accident. There's a mix of languages, cultures, and personalities, making every interaction unique. You witness everything from fear to relief, sometimes in the same room at the same time. Working in the ER is humbling, and it teaches you to see the humanity in all of us.

Triage is essential in the ER, which means you must prioritize patients even when it seems unnatural or makes you feel a bit guilty. It's tough to walk by patients who may be in pain and crying out for help. You can't always stop to comfort someone as you might in other settings because someone else in a more serious condition is counting on you. The patient in excruciating stomach pain may have to wait until you attend to the unresponsive patient with the plummeting blood pressure.

The ER sees it all. Drama comes with the territory, and things don't tend to be calm for any real length of time. Some patients may act out or even harm themselves in their most vulnerable moments. You will often deal with law enforcement, family drama, and other tense situations that remind you of an episode of *Grey's Anatomy*. It's emotionally heavy, but you get through it by focusing on the patient in front of you and what they need.

ER Nurses: The Action-Movie Heroes

Like nursing as a whole, patient care in the ER is challenging but also exceptionally rewarding. You're pushed to your limits, progress quickly, and make an impact every shift. The ER calls for a

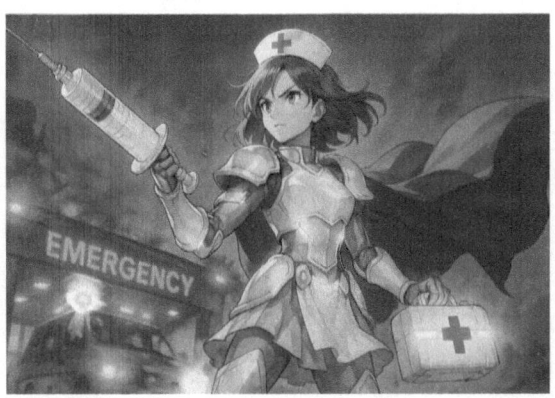

special kind of grit. It's an environment that tests you and shapes you in a way few other departments can.

Intensive Care Unit

The intensive care unit is not for the fainthearted. Here, life and death are in a constant battle for control, with the nurse leading life's charge. Every second can feel like your patience, passion, and perseverance are being tested. Patients here are hanging on by a thread, and every breath and heartbeat matters.

Most ICUs are "general," meaning you'll see a variety of cases that keep you on your toes. It could be a young trauma victim one moment and a post-surgical patient fighting a severe infection the next. These patients are critically ill, hooked up to every machine you can imagine with tubes and wires seeming to fill every inch of the room. You have to be ready for anything because things can change in a second and often do. One minute, you're documenting a set of routine vitals, and the next, you're rushing to respond to a sudden drop in oxygen levels.

The atmosphere itself is electric. There's a constant hum in the ICU, but not from voices. It's the steady beeping of monitors, the mechanical hiss of ventilators, and the soft clicks of IV pumps. It's a symphony of survival. Every sound represents something that is helping to keep your patient alive or alert when things may not be right. Make no mistake: you're not just a nurse; you're a lifeline between a machine and the person it's keeping alive.

> *There's a constant hum in the ICU, but not from voices. It's the steady beeping of monitors, the mechanical hiss of ventilators, and the soft clicks of IV pumps. It's a symphony of survival.*

In the ICU, patients are usually intubated and unresponsive, which means you will probably spend more time communicating with families than with the patients. Families fear the unknown and add a layer of raw emotion to every shift, often focusing on relatively minor things that they are able to control. Don't be surprised to see them fussing because a sock has fallen off the patient's foot and is lying on the floor or they weren't able to visit them at 2:00 in the morning after visiting hours—small transgressions that may not seem critical considering everything else going on with the patient. For you, these concerns may seem trivial, but for them, it's a way of showing love when they feel completely powerless.

ICU Nurses: The Vitals Vigilantes

The ICU offers a particularly intense environment unlike anywhere else in the hospital. If you want to be right in the thick of it, the ICU may be the home you're looking for. The learning curve is fast and steep, and it's often the most intense and consequential a nurse can provide, but if you're drawn to high-energy, life-and-death situations (and aren't afraid to dive in), the ICU could be exactly where you're meant to be. Here, every second, every skill, every alarm, and every breath counts. It's an unforgettable experience and, personally speaking, one of the most challenging, rewarding paths you can take in nursing.

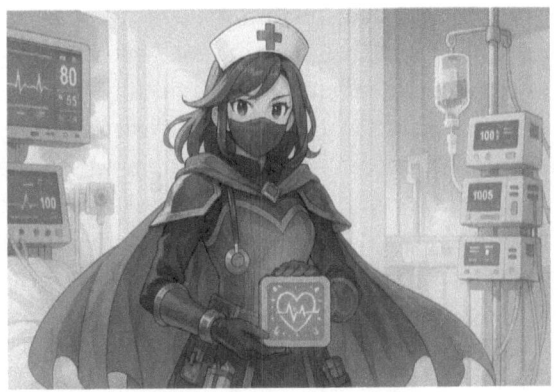

Medical-Surgical

Med-surg units are the unshakeable backbone of hospital nursing, the pulse of patient care. Med-surg is often seen as the "starter" unit, but don't buy into the myth that it's any less demanding than ER or ICU. If anything, this is the battleground where you can build the core skills that will shape your entire nursing career. For those looking to be challenged in ways they never imagined, this is where a heap of real nursing happens.

In med-surg, the variety of patient cases is staggering. You care for people recovering from surgeries, managing long-term chronic conditions, or stabilizing after acute illnesses. Most patients are stable enough to avoid intensive monitoring, but they're by no means "easy." In fact, they're often dealing with a mix of complex health issues. Imagine, for example, a heart condition, diabetes, post-op hip replacement, and early-onset dementia all in one patient. It's a constant exercise in balancing care priorities, adapting quickly, and making sharp clinical decisions. You don't just give meds and check vitals here; you put your knowledge, instincts, and grit to the test every shift.

Keep in mind that med-surg patients are often active participants in their own care. They ask questions, want to be part of the decision-making, and may even challenge you and your competency. It's not uncommon for them to refuse medication or request a change in their plan of care, which keeps you sharp and ready to reeducate them (while respecting their autonomy). It's not just the patients who you will be engaged with. You'll also find that there are med-surg patients who are fortunate enough to have families who are very involved, asking questions, providing information, and wanting to understand everything. They rely on you to guide them through their loved one's recovery, but they can also be helpful to you, which means you're not just treating patients; you're building relationships and educating families too.

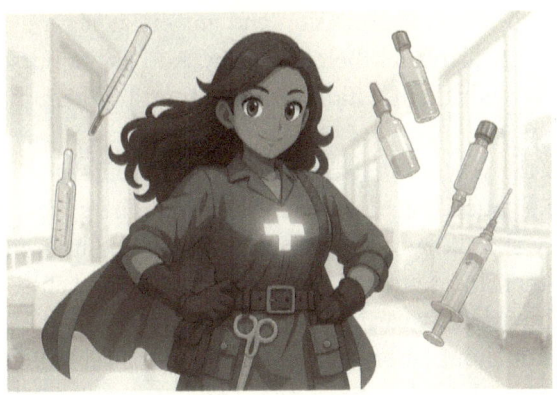

Time management and multitasking are nonnegotiable here. Typically, with four to five patients at a time, you're constantly prioritizing, assessing, and adjusting your plan throughout your shift. This is where your ability to stay organized will make you or break you.

Med-Surg Nurses: The Swiss Army Knives of Nursing

Med-surg nurses are often described as the Swiss Army knives of the nursing world because they can handle pretty much anything. Every shift on a med-surg unit helps nurses hone new skills. This is where you become a well-rounded nurse, with skills that you can use anywhere *if* you choose to explore other areas of nursing. Med-surg may not have the intense drama of an ICU or ER, but it is a demanding and deeply rewarding environment. For nurses who seek variety and the chance to make a meaningful impact every day, med-surg is the ultimate training ground.

Labor and Delivery

Nursing care in L&D is an experience like no other. Imagine walking into work, knowing that you'll be part of one of the biggest moments of a family's life: the birth of a child. L&D is usually buzzing with excitement and anticipation and, like other units, can be filled with tension and anxiety as nervous families anticipate the arrival of their new baby. And as the nurse, you're right there with them, guiding and supporting them every step of the way.

In L&D, you're not just dealing with patients; you're part of something much bigger. Unlike other units, here, you're caring for a very specific group of people: women about to give birth, often in their most vulnerable and emotional moments. And the catch? You are truly caring for two patients: the mother and her baby. Throughout labor, you monitor both closely: the mother's contractions, the baby's heart rate. L&D nurses typically handle one or two sets of patients at a time, allowing for an intense focus on the needs of each family. When mom is having contractions, you're there with a word of support and a hand to squeeze. And though birth is usually a joyful process, the stakes can go from 0 to 100 in minutes and throw you right into the thick of it, helping bring mother and baby through safely.

That's not to say that every patient encounter ends with a happy family headed home with a beautiful, healthy newborn. The truth is, there will always be heartbreaking outcomes: a baby with a congenital birth defect in for a long stay in the NICU, a mother experiencing the stillbirth of her first child, or a new dad faced with the unexpected hardship of taking care of his newborn son after losing his wife during labor. It's essential for nurses considering L&D to be aware that not every outcome will be joyful.

L&D Nurses: The Stork Squad

For nurses who thrive in a dynamic, specialized-care setting, it's hard to imagine anything more gratifying. As an L&D nurse, you're constantly learning and expanding your skills in life-changing ways. If you're looking for a place where each shift brings something unforgettable and you walk away from every day knowing that you've helped create a moment your patient will remember

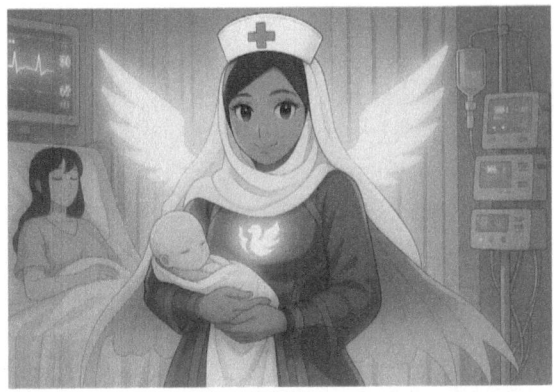

forever, L&D might be your perfect fit. You'll come out of work each day exhausted, maybe even overwhelmed, but with a sense of purpose and satisfaction that few careers can offer.

Oncology

The oncology unit hums with a symphony of soft beeps from IV pumps and the quiet shuffle of slippered feet moving down the hallway. The air carries a faint medicinal tang from disinfectants, blending with the comforting aroma of fresh coffee brewing in the family lounge. This environment feels different from other hospital floor, a little less clinical and a lot more personal. If you peek into the patient rooms, you might see family photos perched on the windowsills, perhaps a colorful quilt draped over the bed, or stuffed animals resting on the nightstand, evidence of the long stays that many patients endure.

Nurses move from the nurses' station to the Pyxis machine and into the patient's room with the muscle memory of a skilled dancer. Pharmacy techs push carts loaded with hazardous medications, gliding quietly across the polished floors. A nurse dons gloves and a shapeless, yellow gown, carefully handling a bag of chemotherapy drugs. The bright yellow label, marked with warnings, serves as a constant reminder of the precision and attention to detail required. Every action is deliberate—adjusting infusion rates, double-checking dosages, documenting every detail.

Many conversations in departments such as oncology carry a distinctly heavier weight than in other areas of the hospital. In one room, a nurse sits beside the bed, her voice low and soothing as she explains to her 72-year-old male patient how the toxic infusion she's about to administer will make him feel worse before he gets better. The patient nods, eyes scanning the printed information in the nurse's hand with an expression of quiet apprehension and calm determination. At the end of the hall, the charge nurse leans against the doorway, laughing with a patient whose head is wrapped in a brightly colored scarf. The genuine laughter is a short-lived escape as the team awaits the results from yesterday's scan to see if the tumor has shrunk. Emotion runs deep in this space. In the family lounge, a nurse claps joyfully with his patient's husband and daughter after hearing the news of remission, tearful smiles brightening the unit like sunlight. The same nurse will end his shift embracing a grieving mother, silently acknowledging the heartbreaking loss of her only son.

> The oncology unit is a place of profound connection. Nurses are more than caregivers. They are companions alongside their patients in the fight of their lives.

Education is everywhere, all the time, with every patient and family member. Nurses patiently explain how chemotherapy might cause nausea, why hydration is critical, or how to manage fatigue. Social workers and chaplains are virtually omnipresent to help the nurses and doctors support patients and family members navigating the implications of their medical conditions. At the center of the care team, the nurse is the coordinator of all the care the patient needs.

Oncology Nurses: The Soulful Warriors

The nurses in oncology are more than merely the providers of clinical care. They are truly challenged to have a 360-degree

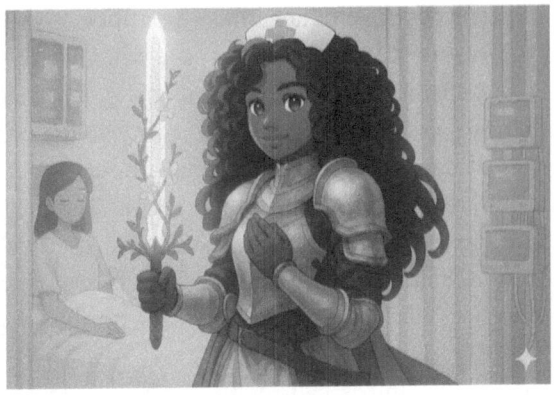

approach to meeting the patient's needs. Clinician, advocate, educator—the nurse is a bridge between complex medical jargon and human understanding. The oncology unit is a place of profound connection. Nurses are more than caregivers. They are companions alongside their patients in the fight of their lives.

Behavioral Health

The behavioral health unit has a special rhythm that is difficult to describe unless you've been there. For safety purposes, there are usually two sets of doors with separate secure entrances. The act of badging to get through one set of doors and waiting for those doors to close before you can badge yourself in from the anteroom onto the actual unit can be both reassuring and unsettling. The air feels different here: charged, like a summer thunderstorm waiting to unleash a series of lightning strikes. The walls are free from decor, and the hallways are wide and uncluttered, designed to promote both safety and a sense of openness free of unintentional emotional triggers. Despite the peaceful aesthetic, there's a palpable tension, a quiet readiness among the staff, who move with purpose yet remain watchful.

The design of the unit reflects the delivery of care. From the moment the day begins, every structured activity has its place, providing patients with a predictability that supports their stability. Breakfast is served in a common space where some patients sit quietly, lost in thought, while others chat softly. Medication rounds are next, a systematic process to improve the chances of successful treatment for patients experiencing an emotional or mental health crisis. Nurses offer gentle encouragement to those who hesitate. In the therapy room, patients sit in a welcoming circle with soft chairs. Later in the day, some of the patients will be encouraged to play card games or work on jigsaw puzzles, while others seek refuge in their rooms.

Most days, the unit is calm with minimal drama. But that calm is delicate. A sudden outburst can ripple through the unit like a pebble skipping across still waters. De-escalation is not just a skill in behavioral health; it's an art.

Every patient interaction is a chance to connect, to build trust when patients are often at their most vulnerable. The challenges these patients face go beyond their DSM-IV diagnoses. Many have suffered physical and emotional abuse, don't have stable housing, struggle with substance abuse, or don't have strong personal relationships. Behavioral-health nurses become both caregivers and anchors, offering steady guidance in moments of chaos. They listen with an intensity that goes beyond words,

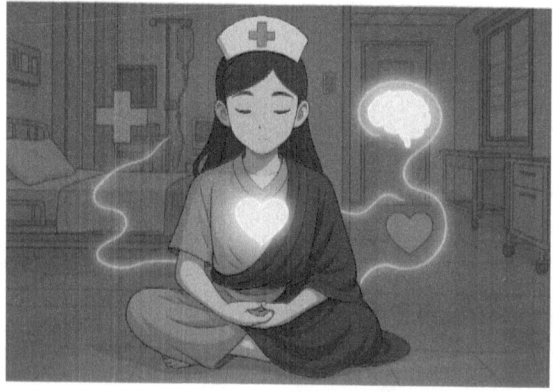

catching the quiet despair behind a patient's bravado or the hope buried under layers of fear.

Behavioral-Health Nurses: The Zen Masters

This environment requires compassion, composure, and human-interaction skills that sharpen with each shift. It's not easy, but it's profoundly rewarding. For new nurses, this is a place where you grow fast, learning to navigate not just the storm but also the moments of quiet hope that follow. This is where mental crisis meets human connection, and every day brings the chance to help someone find their way back to stability.

Operating Room

Stepping into the operating room is an otherworldly experience. Overhead lights illuminate the space with a harsh radiance designed to focus everyone's attention on the sterile field and the patient where all the action happens. From the surgical instruments to the array of machines, from the metallic tables to the polished floors, the OR is beyond sterile.

In this intensely organized atmosphere, every person has a specific job, and they're all hyper-focused on their role. The surgeon stands at the center of it all, hands working with calm precision, while the scrub nurse stands at the ready, prepared to hand off instruments at just the right moment (a role increasingly being performed by a surgical tech). Outside the sterile field, the circulating nurse moves around the room, grabbing supplies, adjusting equipment, and coordinating with activities outside the OR. There's less multitasking than in the units, intentionally, because every action has a purpose, and there's no room for distractions.

The sounds of the OR are much calmer and composed than on the floor. Depending on the procedure, you may hear the clip of scissors, the mechanical whirring and clicks of the surgical robot, or the literal hammering during a knee replacement. In the background, music plays—anything from classical music to rock and roll—whatever the surgeon chooses to keep the surgical team focused yet composed. Absent are the ringing phones, squeaky carts, beeping call lights, and constant chatter of the inpatient units.

The procedural dance in the OR is a well-rehearsed routine, where every detail matters to keep patients safe. That said, the intensity in the room can skyrocket in an instant. One second, the procedure is going smoothly and according to plan; the next, the sound of a critical alarm cuts through the air and everything changes. It's the nurse in the OR who plays the critical role of maintaining a sense of calm and making sure the team is prepared to get the patient safely through the procedure.

OR Nurses: The Directors of the Dance

The OR is, at times, like an impromptu dance, and that's also what makes it so unique. It's not just about excitement; it's about the team's trust and focus that allows them to care for the patient, one deliberate move after another. For those who thrive on intensity and purpose, the OR is where it all comes together. Whether you are the scrub nurse maintaining the sterile field with the surgical team or the circulating nurse coordinating all the action

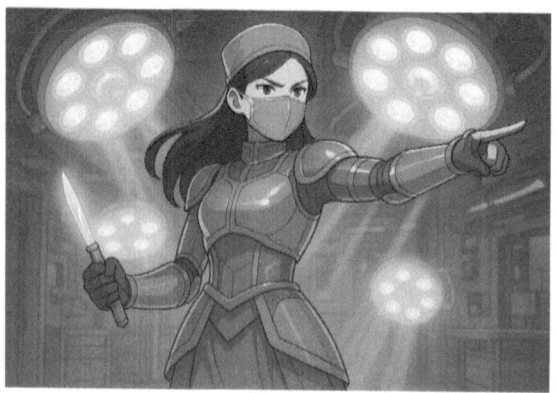

inside and outside the OR, the phrase "keep calm and carry on" may have been created just for you.

> **POWER PLAY:** Ask yourself, "Do I thrive in high-pressure situations, or do I prefer a steady, methodical pace? Am I drawn to hands-on procedures, or do I find fulfillment in long-term patient connections?"

Vibe Check Complete—You've Got This!

Finding your unit vibe isn't just about choosing a job. It's about choosing an environment where you can thrive. When your personality and work style align with your unit, the long shifts feel more rewarding, and you grow both as a nurse and as a person. But remember: finding the right fit is a journey.

How do you figure out where you truly belong? It starts with looking inward. Your strengths, preferences, and work style play a huge role in determining which unit will bring out your best.

In the next chapter, we dive into self-assessment, helping you uncover what makes you tick as a nurse so you can confidently step into the unit that fits you best.

CHAPTER 2

Personality Self-Assessment

The famous Greek philosopher Aristotle has been quoted as saying, "Knowing yourself is the beginning of all wisdom." Now that we've explored what makes different hospital units unique, let's invoke the spirit of the great Greek thinker and shift the focus to you. After all, during your first year as a nurse, you'll have spent over 2,500 hours working in your chosen department (not even counting overtime!). You deserve the best chance to succeed and thrive in an environment that aligns with your natural tendencies and skill set.

Ask yourself this: "Do I want to start my nursing career in a department where I rarely use my natural strengths and spend every shift struggling with new skills I don't have yet or maybe don't even want to develop? Or would I rather work in a department where I feel confident because I am regularly using my natural talents every shift while growing new skills over time?"

I know which option sounds better to me, and maybe you agree. I would rather have a plan to pick a unit that complements my natural skills and talents. One that pushes me to continue to grow and hone new skills and talents and not leave it to chance.

This chapter outlines a few personality-assessment tools you can use to help objectively identify the strengths that come naturally to you. One of my favorite thought leaders is Simon Sinek, a leadership expert, author, and speaker known for his "Start with

Why" concept.[v] So before we review the actual tools, let's discuss *why* (pun intended) this matters to the career and life you've worked so hard to build.

Ask yourself this: "Do I want to start my nursing career in a department where I rarely use my natural strengths and spend every shift struggling with new skills I don't have yet or maybe don't even want to develop? Or would I rather work in a department where I feel confident because I am regularly using my natural talents every shift while growing new skills over time?"

We All Have Different Superpowers

To illustrate this point, let's look at a comparison from the sport of track and field (bear with me; I promise this is going somewhere!).

When I took Anatomy and Physiology 1 in nursing school, we studied a case about the physiological differences between long-distance runners such as marathoners and cross-country athletes and sprinters who dominate such events as the 100-meter dash. Here's the thing: long-distance runners are naturally equipped with an abundance of slow-twitch muscle fibers, which contract slowly but can sustain effort for long periods. On the flip side, sprinters rely on fast-twitch muscle fibers, which contract quickly and explosively. Now, that doesn't mean someone with predominantly slow-twitch muscles can't train to be faster or more explosive. Of course they can. It would just take them more effort and time to develop those fast-twitch fibers.

Similarly, as a nurse, you have your own unique strengths. Doesn't it make sense to start your career by putting your best foot forward, feeling confident and resilient, leaning on the strengths and abilities that come naturally and from there, building on and refining other skills over time?

Mismatch Can Lead to Burnout

Burnout, defined as emotional exhaustion, depersonalization, and reduced personal accomplishment, is an unfortunate reality in the nursing profession.[vi] There has been a lot of talk about burnout in recent years, but what does it have to do with what we are talking about here? A mismatch between a nurse's inherent traits and their role can, and often does, lead to increased stress and emotional exhaustion. Studies show that misalignments between the work environment and a nurse's personality characteristics contribute to higher rates of burnout.[vii] This not only affects a nurse's health but can also lead to decreased quality of patient care and patient satisfaction.

Research also shows that aligning personalities and natural strengths to the work environment not only promotes mental

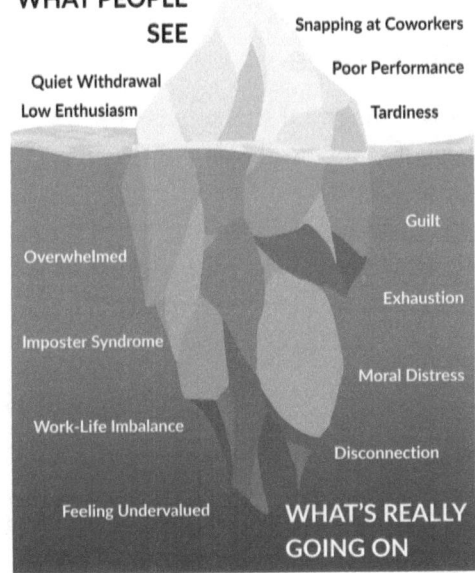

wellness but also boosts confidence. When nurses feel competent and supported in their roles, they are more likely to engage positively with patients and colleagues, leading to a more fulfilling career.[viii] Leaning into these traits can also help minimize the risk of "imposter syndrome," a psychological experience where individuals doubt their abilities and fear being exposed as frauds.[ix] Studies show that imposter syndrome can lead to anxiety, burnout, and lower job satisfaction.[x]

Carefully considering how your personal attributes align with your nursing unit can prevent burnout, enhance job satisfaction, and promote overall well-being. Your desire to go on this journey of self-discovery will pay off tremendously as you make moves to avoid the stressors that may negatively impact your nursing career. Now, let me make sure I emphasize that we aren't talking about how smart someone is or how well they did in nursing school. We are taking into consideration your personality traits that have been at the essence of who you are from the day you took your first breath.

Personality Tests

The first step to aligning your strengths is using a personality test. There are many of them out there, and they tend to vary based on their purpose. Tests to evaluate love and relationships, communication styles, and career planning are just a few examples. The following are a few of my favorite personality-testing options that have been found to align well with career planning. In no way is this an endorsement of one over any other. Ultimately, it is whatever works for *you!*

CliftonStrengths®

CliftonStrengths is a self-assessment that identifies a small set of your most prominent personal talents from a broader collection of possible themes. The idea is that when you understand and intentionally use your strongest traits, you can improve your performance, decision-making, and satisfaction in both personal and professional settings. The official version provides a ranked list of your top talents and guidance on how to apply them. Based on Gallup research and positive psychology from Donald Clifton, CliftonStrengths is all about focusing on what makes you shine instead of on what you need to "fix."[xi] Gallup's research highlights the significant impact of strengths-based employee development on engagement and performance including the following key findings:[xii]

- Employees who utilize their strengths daily are nearly six times more engaged at work.
- Organizations implementing strengths-based development report increases of 10 to 19 percent in sales and 14 to 29 percent in profit.
- Employees who feel that their strengths are utilized are less likely to leave their company.

Why it matters for choosing a nursing unit

Knowing your natural talents can help you choose a unit where those strengths are valued and needed. For example, if you excel at building trust quickly, you might thrive in patient-centered units like oncology or pediatrics.

Myers-Briggs Type Indicator® (MBTI®)

The Myers-Briggs Type Indicator is a personality tool that groups people into 16 personality types based on four preference pairs: how you focus your attention, how you take in information, how you make decisions, and how you approach the outside world. It is designed to help people better understand their communication styles, work preferences, and ways of interacting with others. The MBTI assessment is a fun and fascinating way to uncover both your personality type and how you see the world.[xiii]

Why it matters for choosing a nursing unit:
Your MBTI type can guide you toward units that align with how you like to work. If you are energized by fast decision-making and constant change, a critical-care unit may be a better match than a slower-paced specialty.

DISC

The DISC assessment categorizes behavioral tendencies into four main styles: dominance, influence, steadiness, and conscientiousness. It focuses on how you approach tasks, challenges, and relationships, making it a useful tool for improving communication, resolving conflicts, and building stronger teams. Research shows that DISC can be great for understanding how you engage with patients, families, and colleagues.[xiv]

Why it matters for choosing a nursing unit:
Understanding your DISC style can help you find a team culture that fits. A dominance-heavy style might do well in a high-pressure environment like the emergency department, whereas a steadiness style may prefer predictable, relationship-focused settings.

Five-Factor Model (OCEAN)

The Five-Factor Model, often remembered by the acronym OCEAN, measures personality across five broad traits: openness, conscientiousness, extraversion, agreeableness, and neuroticism. It is widely used in psychology to describe personality in a way that is both scientifically grounded and easy to relate to real-world behavior.

Why it matters for choosing a nursing unit:
Your scores can help you understand where you will feel most comfortable and effective. A nurse high in openness may enjoy a unit with evolving technology and protocols, whereas a nurse high in conscientiousness may thrive in units that require strict adherence to procedures.

How to Use the Tests—Without Overthinking It

As you can see, these tools share common descriptors, but they are also unique. What happens if you get mixed results after taking more than one assessment? Congratulations! It means that, like most people, you have more than one strength. The key is to determine which strength is most important to you or which is the most dominant by looking for patterns across multiple tests.

POWER PLAY: Scan this QR code for a worksheet that will help you track your test results and determine your best fit.

Personality Assessment Worksheet

https://auspicious-water-67783.myflodesk.com/assessmentworksheet

> *What is the thing that's going to make you wake up, crawl out of bed, leave your family, and be on your feet for the majority of a 12-hour shift? Whatever that trait is, that's the one you prioritize!*

Another tip for interpreting mixed results is to evaluate your strongest superpowers. Let's pretend that you are a superhero with the ability to fly, read people's minds, and see in the dark. More than anything, you love to fly, and it's one of your top superpowers. And since you don't always want to know what other people are thinking and hardly ever have the need to see in the dark, you would prioritize flying. It's the same with these assessment results. You would make the determination based on what is more important to you. Remember: this is about *you*, not about the test! What is the thing that's going to make you wake up, crawl out of bed, leave your family, and be on your feet for the majority of a 12-hour shift? Whatever that trait is, that's the one you prioritize!

In the following chapters, we explore the unique dynamics of each unit to help you discover where your strengths and passions fit in best. But beyond the setting, nursing is also about how it feels—the rhythm of the work, the emotional investment, and the connections you build. To start, let's consider the pace, because finding the right environment begins with understanding the energy and flow that truly suit you best.

CHAPTER 3

Consider the Pace

Salsa, Shaku Shaku, swing, Bharatanatyam, or ballet. There are literally hundreds of dances, reflecting music genres and cultures from all around the globe. Different types of dances are primarily based on the rhythm and accompanying movements of that dance style. I recall being in the third grade when we did a ballet to hip-hop music and tap danced to Mozart. The point of doing so was to learn that the primary thing that differentiates one dance style from another is the rhythm and pace of the music, very similar to nursing units. The chaotic pace and energy in the ED are obvious as soon as you enter through those double doors, just as the deliberate calm of the oncology unit has its own intensity. It's more than just evaluating how fast things move. It's about finding the rhythm that suits YOU. Think of nursing as a dance, with each unit moving to its own beat. So how do you choose the right tempo?

This chapter emphasizes why the pace of a unit is important and how it impacts your job satisfaction and how engaged you are in your daily work. Then it explains why it's important to consider the personality traits you may have that align with the pace. Let's dive in!

Note: Throughout this book, I share real stories. Some are from nurses I've interviewed; others were swapped over chips, salsa, and maybe a margarita or two. These are the kinds of stories that stick with you—the kind we tell each other after long shifts or in group texts that start with, "Girl, you won't believe…"

All names have been changed, either to protect patient privacy or because someone said, "Please don't let my mama read this."

Stacie's Story

I still remember the moment I finally felt like I was at home in the ED. The chime of the ambulance radio snapped me out of my focus. I'd only been on shift for two hours, but I'd already treated everything from sprained ankles to a massive stroke. Six months ago, I was a brand-new nurse, jumping into every call with a mix of nerves and excitement. Now, adrenaline was just part of my routine, fueling me as the controlled chaos of the emergency department charged on.

"Level 1…GSW coming in!" someone yelled, and I was off, heart pounding as I rushed to prep the trauma bay for a gunshot victim. This was the ER, where time isn't on anyone's side.

I glanced at my current patient, an older guy with chest pain who looked up at me, wide-eyed and nervous. "You're in good hands," I said, handing him off to another nurse before sprinting toward the trauma bay.

The paramedics wheeled in a young guy, maybe in his mid-20s, his face pale and covered in sweat. His shirt was soaked in blood around a gunshot wound high on his left side. I locked eyes with the paramedic for a second as he gave the rundown.

"Single gunshot wound to the upper abdomen. BP's dropping; last check was 90 over 60, heart rate 140."

I nodded, sliding into place as my team closed in around him. Monitors beeped in warning as I adjusted his IV line and started another for fluids. He gasped for breath, eyes darting around in panic. I leaned close, trying to catch his attention.

"Hey, you're safe here. We're going to take care of you."

My words barely left my mouth before orders flew around us—labs, fluids, pain meds, trauma consult, get a surgeon on standby, stat chest X-ray. The attending physician started working on the wound, hands moving fast and sure. I watched the monitors, my mind keeping time with the beeping, each second ticking faster than it should.

> *In the middle of it all, it hit me that I wasn't that brand-new nurse anymore, wondering if I was going to like working in the ER, if I was going to succeed. I loved everything about working here, from the adrenaline rush and having to always think fast on my feet to going with my gut, often without a second guess. The next patient was already on their way through the doors, but I was ready and couldn't wait to see what was in store for me next.*

Why Does the Pace Matter?

The pace of a unit depends on a few key things: patient volume, turnover, acuity, and the unit's focus. High-turnover units such as the ER and med-surg are often busy, with more patients coming and going than in other hospital departments. These units usually have higher nurse-to-patient ratios, which means you're managing more people. On the flip side, ICU nurses typically have fewer patients but need to stay laser-focused because the stakes are higher, requiring quick, critical decisions.

Specialized areas also bring their own rhythms. Labor and delivery, for instance, can shift from calm to chaos in seconds with emergencies or unscheduled births. In contrast, units such as palliative care or behavioral health often have slower paces, emphasizing thoughtful, longer interactions. Oncology nursing is another example of where the pace can be slower but deeply personal, building long-term relationships with patients.

> *... let's consider the regretful necessity of housekeeping. I am completely capable of cleaning my home and think I do a pretty good job, but you couldn't pay me any amount of money to spend 12 hours a day, 3 days a week doing it!*

Here's the thing: the pace you thrive in doesn't define your intelligence or knowledge. I've heard nursing students say things like, "I have a 4.0 GPA and crushed pharmacology, so I'll do great in the ICU because I think fast on my feet."

I don't know where this assumption comes from—maybe nursing school, that new show *The Pitt*, or just public perception. "I'm smart" *equals* "I think quickly on my feet" *equals* "I should be working in the ER or ICU." I don't know who came up with this, but it's just not true. To illustrate this point outside of nursing, let's consider the regretful necessity of housekeeping. I am completely capable of cleaning my home and think I do a pretty good job, but you couldn't pay me any amount of money to spend 12 hours a day, 3 days a week doing it! Grades don't decide where you'll feel comfortable or what you'll find fulfilling. Instead, think about how you prefer to process information and make decisions. Be real with yourself about what pace fits your personality.

For example, imagine working in the ED when a 65-year-old male comes in unresponsive after experiencing chest pains. You get an order to give a nitrate. You know the five rights of medication administration and that nitrates are contraindicated for patients on erectile-dysfunction meds. Are you comfortable giving that med without knowing his medication history? Or would you prefer a setting where you have time to review all home medications and double-check for interactions? It's not about being smart; it's about whether you're comfortable in the moment.

Keep in mind that just because you *can* handle a situation doesn't mean you want to spend every shift doing that. Find the pace that works for *you*. It's about what you *want* to do in addition to what you *can* do.

Why should you care about the pace and rhythm in your chosen department? Picture this: You're halfway through your very first nursing shift. The phone is constantly ringing, alarms are beeping, you're getting pulled in five different directions, and you haven't had a chance to breathe in what feels like hours. Or imagine the opposite: you're on a unit where things are steady and calm and you get to know your patients on a deeper level. The pace of a unit can be the difference between loving your nursing life and feeling overwhelmed.

Which pace do you like better? What did your personality assessment(s) tell you about yourself? What are your strengths? Do you love the rush of adrenaline, or do you prefer a more methodical, thoughtful approach to your work? Choosing the right pace is crucial because it's directly tied to how you'll feel at the end of the day: energized and fulfilled or completely drained.

Matching Your Personality to the Pace

Fast-Paced Units

As we talked about in chapter 1, working in a fast-paced nursing unit such as the ER, ICU, or L&D isn't for everyone, but if you're someone who loves a challenge, thrives under pressure, and gets energized by action, it might be exactly where you belong. These environments move fast, and they require a certain set of traits to succeed. Let's break down what makes a great nurse in these high-energy settings:

- You are an adrenaline junkie.

  In fast-paced units, things can go from 0 to 100 in a heartbeat. You need to be able to make decisions on the spot, trust your instincts, and prioritize tasks without hesitation. If you're the kind of person who stays sharp under pressure and likes figuring things out quickly, this is a skill that will help you crush it in a fast-moving environment.

- You can go with the flow.

  One thing about fast-paced units: no two shifts are ever the same. Maybe you planned to chart but a patient crashes, or you thought you'd finally grab lunch but an ambulance just pulled up with three critical patients. If you're adaptable and good at pivoting when things don't go as planned, you'll feel right at home.

- You're a strong communicator.

    SBAR, SBAR, SBAR! Situation. Background. Assessment. Recommendation. Our favorite communication tool is important in any care setting but is essential in units where time is critical in the struggle between life and death. In the fast-paced unit, a strong ability to communicate effectively with an emphasis on prioritizing critical information is a must. Whether it's giving a quick but clear update to a doctor or calming a patient's family in the middle of a crisis, how you communicate can make or break a situation. Nurses who thrive in these environments are great at staying calm, being direct, and making sure everyone is on the same page even when it feels like the world is spinning around them.

- You keep cool under pressure.

    Let's be real. Working in a fast-paced unit can get intense. Things happen fast and emotions can run high. Nurses who excel here are the ones who keep their cool, focus on the task at hand, and bring a sense of calm to the chaos. If you're the friend everyone calls when they're freaking out because they know you'll handle it, this might be your thing.

- You love to be the problem-solver.

    Fast-paced units don't leave much room for, "Let me think about that and get back to you." You must solve problems quickly and think critically, whether it's figuring out why a patient's condition is deteriorating or troubleshooting equipment in the middle of a code. If you love working through challenges and finding solutions, this is a skill you'll use every day.

- You're driven and love a good challenge.

    Fast-paced units are not easy. Long hours, constant action, and heavy workloads can be exhausting. But if you're motivated by the feeling of accomplishment and love being in the middle of the action, this environment can be incredibly rewarding. Nurses who thrive here are the ones who feel proud of handling whatever a shift throws at them.

If you're the kind of person who thrives on energy, loves a challenge, and enjoys working with a fast-moving team, a fast-paced unit could be the perfect fit. But if you're not quite feeling it, that's okay too!

Slower-Paced Units

Slower-paced units have their own unique rewards.

Working in a slower-paced nursing unit such as rehab, palliative care, oncology, or long-term care offers a completely different experience than the high-speed hustle of the ER or ICU. These environments are more focused on steady workflows, building meaningful relationships, and providing long-term, thoughtful care. If you're wondering whether this might be your fit, here are some key traits that help nurses thrive in these settings:

- You have patience and empathy.

  Slower-paced units often involve caring for patients over extended periods, allowing you to form deeper connections. Nurses who are naturally patient and compassionate excel here. If you're someone who finds fulfillment in really getting to know your patients and supporting them emotionally, this kind of environment is a great match.

- You are calm and dependable.

  Patients in these units often face chronic illnesses, long recoveries, or end-of-life care. Being a calm, dependable presence helps build trust and provides comfort for patients and families. If you're steady under pressure and good at creating a peaceful environment, you'll bring a sense of stability to the unit.

- You love structure and routine.

  Though no nursing job is ever completely predictable, slower-paced units tend to have more routine workflows compared with the unpredictability of fast-paced environments. Nurses who prefer structure and consistency will feel right at home in these settings.

If you're someone who values meaningful relationships, enjoys taking time to focus on the details, and finds satisfaction in creating a calm, supportive atmosphere, a slower-paced unit might be perfect for you. These environments give you the chance to make a lasting impact, not just in your patients' care but also in their overall experience. And if this doesn't sound like your vibe? No worries! There's a nursing role out there that will fit your strengths and help you thrive.

> **POWER PLAY:** Post-Clinical Pulse Check
> After every clinical shift, rate these three things:
> 1. How mentally exhausted are you?
> 2. Did you feel overstimulated or bored?
> 3. Would you want to do this three days in a row?
>
> Simple. Quick. But when you track it over time, patterns show up. That's data, baby! Use it to make your next move.

Is This Your Fit?

Where do you see yourself in all this? Are you the decision-maker, the motivator, the calm force, or the detail master? Here's the thing: fast-paced units need a mix of all these traits. Maybe you see yourself in one of them, or maybe you're a combo of a few. Nursing is full of opportunities, and there are plenty of units where the pace is slower, more methodical, and just as important. The key is to figure out what feels right for you. After all, the best nurses aren't all in the ICU or in the palliative-care unit. The best nurses are the ones who find a rhythm that fits their own personality so that they are in the best position to continue to learn and build on the skills they haven't fully developed.

The world of nursing is wide, and every unit dances to its own beat. Whether you thrive on the thrill of the fast-paced or find peace in a slower rhythm, there's a place for you. Trust your instincts and you'll know when you've found the right rhythm for your career. So lace up your shoes, feel the pulse, and find the pace that allows you to love what you do.

Now, nursing isn't just about finding the right environment. It's about the emotional investment that comes with caring for others. The connections you form, the challenges you face, and the passion you pour into your work will shape your journey just as much as the setting you choose will. That's what we'll dive into next.

CHAPTER 4

Emotional Investment

Let's be honest. Hospitals are emotional pressure cookers. You may be surrounded by people having one of their worst (or best!) days ever. The 65-year-old clutching his chest in the ED? He's petrified that he's having a heart attack. That first-time mom in L&D? She's scared but hopeful her firstborn will be healthy. They are both relying on complete strangers to help them in their most vulnerable moments. In any care setting, there will be storms of emotions, and guess who's right in the middle of it? You...us... nurses! Think about it: no matter where you seek care in the hospital, there will be a nurse providing it.

In this chapter, we explore why considering your emotional investment is so important. Then we examine the emotional investment associated with various departments and unpack how your personality traits and natural strengths may align. Do you find it rewarding to be in the thick of all the emotions and connect naturally with others during stressful times? Or do you find that making deep emotional connections with people you don't really know is not a primary source of fulfillment at work? Understanding these preferences isn't just about job satisfaction. It's about creating a sustainable career in which

> *In any care setting, there will be storms of emotions, and guess who's right in the middle of it? You...us... nurses! Think about it: no matter where you seek care in the hospital, there will be a nurse providing it.*

you can maintain your emotional well-being while providing excellent patient care. Let's get into it!

Amaya's Anecdote

I took a shaky breath as I stepped onto the pediatrics floor with my clinical instructor. I could feel the tension building in my neck and shoulders. I'd been nervous before, but I had never felt apprehension like this. This was different. It was my first pediatric clinical rotation as a nursing student, and it was on the pediatric oncology floor. I had two little ones myself, three and five years old, and as I watched them playing together the day before, I couldn't help but think to myself that I wouldn't know how to handle it if either of them ever got seriously sick.

The antiseptic smell that permeated the hallway reminded me of countless doctors' visits with my own children. But it was more than the smell. The quiet there felt heavy, broken only by the occasional beeping of monitors and hushed conversations behind closed doors.

My instructor grabbed a chart and told me to review the admission notes.

Lily Carter. Three years old. History of brain cancer. Readmitted for persistent headaches, dizziness, and falls.

As a nursing student, I didn't know that much about pediatrics or cancer, but I had a bad feeling in the pit of my stomach.

"The cancer has probably come back," confirmed my clinical instructor.

It was even worse than that. As I read through the physician notes, I discovered that the cancer was not only back but even more aggressive than before. The tumor was growing and moving down Lily's spinal column. Before I could process this information, I realized from the notes that today the team would be meeting with the parents to let them know that the tumor was inoperable.

My hands trembled slightly as I flipped through the pages, trying to focus on the medical terminology instead of where my brain was pulling me, imagining what these parents must be going through. The floor felt like it was swaying beneath my feet as I found myself thinking about my own children, probably strapped into their car seats in the back of our minivan, singing songs from Barney & Friends with my husband on their way to daycare at that very moment. I could almost hear their cheerful chatter about what snacks they liked the best in after-school care, completely unaware of how fortunate they were to be healthy. They were my whole life, just as Lily was to her parents, and I held back tears at the thought of them having to face what Lily was experiencing.

Get it together, Amaya, I thought to myself. Lily's nurse patted me on my back, giving me a sympathetic look, as if she heard my thoughts. She handed me a pink plastic pitcher full of ice water.

"This will never get easy," she said. "Why don't you go ahead and introduce yourself and take this into them?"

I walked stiffly down the hallway adorned with brightly painted walls displaying smiling jungle animals; the playful cartoon monkeys, giraffes, and elephants were a contradiction to the profound sadness I was feeling. I paused outside the room, taking a couple of deep breaths. How would I handle being in these parents' shoes? The thought made my chest tighten up.

I knocked softly before stepping inside.

I couldn't completely make out faces in the dark room. But I immediately heard Lily start crying softly, "No more. No more. I want to go home."

Her dad got up off the couch, where her mom was sleeping, and went to her. He shushed her and told her that it was okay and that they would be going home soon. The sound of her tiny, frail voice, so tired and scared, pierced right through my professional façade. I watched as her father stroked her hair, his movements gentle but uncertain, as if he were afraid of causing more pain.

I couldn't hold it in. I told them my name quickly and that I was going to rinse out the water pitcher, which I held onto tightly as I rushed to the bathroom. I turned on the faucet and let the cascade of gushing water drown out the sound of me crying.

By the time I'd collected myself and come back into the room, Lily's mom had woken up and opened the curtains. Now in the light of day, I could see the weariness and anxiety written all over their faces. I went to Lily and told her that I would be helping to take care of her. She shyly confessed to me that she missed her big sister and was ready to go home. I wanted to say something reassuring, but nothing felt right. I hadn't quite figured out how to navigate these conversations but knew deep down it would never be easy.

The morning light streaming through the window caught the metallic gleam of the medical equipment surrounding her bed. The room was decorated with crayon drawings and get-well cards, a heartbreaking attempt to make this sterile space feel more like home.

Just then, there was a knock on the door and a team of doctors, the nurse, and a few others, including the chaplain, slowly trudged into the small room. These were the people who had come to tell Lily's parents that their worst nightmare had come true.

I swallowed hard and pulled a handful of stickers from my pocket. "Pick as many as you want."

Lily grabbed a rainbow sticker, sparkling with glitter and neon colors, looked up at me, and gave me a big, crooked smile.

It was at this moment, looking at this precious little girl, that I realized that I couldn't do this.

I couldn't come home to my own babies after days like this, pretending that I hadn't just watched another mother's heartbreak. I wouldn't be able to leave these kids at the hospital and not take their stories and their sorrows home with me. That was my personal decision, and it made me have even more respect for the work that pediatric nurses do.

I just knew that pediatrics wasn't right for me.

> *Walking out of that hospital at the end of my rotation, I felt both lighter and heavier. Lighter because I'd finally admitted the truth to myself, but heavier with the knowledge of what families like Lily's face every day. The afternoon sun felt almost offensive in its brightness, and I found myself imagining Lily standing in the light next to her big sister, its warm rays shining down on her sweet face.*

The Stuff We Don't Chart

Though we're all capable of providing emotional support (it's literally in our job description), not all of us thrive in the same emotional environments. And that's 100 percent okay! It's like choosing between a spring break partying at Señor Frog's in Cancún or one at a private beach with a few friends: both are valid vacation spots, but you might have a strong preference for one over the other.

Nurses are in the business of caring, and emotional connectedness comes with the territory. According to the American Nurses Association, nursing is defined as "the protection, promotion, and optimization of health and abilities, prevention of illness and injury, facilitation of healing, alleviation of suffering through the diagnosis and treatment of human response, and advocacy in the care of individuals, families, groups, communities, and populations."[xv] In order to provide quality nursing, there is a level of emotion involved when caring for another human being.

But let's keep it real. This constant emotional engagement, though rewarding, can take its toll in the form of "compassion fatigue," which is a unique form of burnout that affects healthcare workers who repeatedly bear witness to others' trauma and suffering.[xvi] Think of it like an emotional bank account from which you're constantly making withdrawals (giving empathy and support to patients and families) but not always making enough deposits (self-care and emotional replenishment). Over time, this imbalance can lead to emotional exhaustion, decreased empathy, and a diminished ability to cope with workplace stressors, all of which can lead you down the predictable path toward burnout.

Recognizing and managing compassion fatigue is crucial for a future-proof nursing career.

Back to that emotional bank account: some nurses might find that certain high-intensity units drain their emotional reserves faster than in other hospital units. This isn't a reflection of their caring ability—it's about understanding their own emotional capacity and work environment fit.

I can't say that I have ever met or worked with a nurse who was not capable or willing to deal with the emotional aspects of patient care. However, I have met and worked with nurses who were uncomfortable or did not feel fulfilled when faced with emotionally charged situations. There's no doubt about it: certain departments tend to experience particularly intense and frequent occurrences of high emotions. Consider Amaya's story at the beginning of the chapter. It's not that she was hard-hearted or didn't care. The emotional investment on the pediatric oncology floor was not going to work for her; it pushed her past her limit. This goes back to what I shared earlier. Just because you *can* do it doesn't mean you *want* to, day in and day out...and that's totally fine.

Highly Emotionally Charged Departments

We've already established that providing care for others means that you will inevitably bear witness to trauma and suffering, regardless of the setting. However, there are certain departments in a hospital where the occurrence and level of trauma and suffering witnessed are different. In one department, there is an unexpected battle between life and death played out on every shift. In another, there might be a chronic mental illness that has become an acute crisis. They're all different.

Emotional Investment

Units such as the ED, ICU, oncology, and behavioral health tend to require a level of emotional resilience not common in other departments. In the ED, patient acuity, violence, interpersonal conflict, and mass-casualty incidents are contributing factors. In the ICU and oncology departments, nurses build relationships with patients and families who are facing their very mortality, exposing nurses to prolonged emotional stress. Further, nurses in behavioral-health units consistently address the needs of patients who are usually experiencing a mental crisis that can only be resolved through intimate, personal connections.

If your personality assessment indicates that you are fulfilled by deep connections, you will probably find true fulfillment from the emotional investment in these departments. Think of it as your superpower: you get energized by those deeper patient relationships instead of being drained by them. You may find that the emotional connections in these departments fill your cup, which can help you withstand the impact of witnessing human suffering. Likewise, if you used the OCEAN model, and conscientiousness and agreeableness measures were high, these high-emotion departments are likely right up your alley.

Reality check: you may find it extremely fulfilling to work in the middle of the "ocean of emotions," but you still need to make sure you have enough compassion to give to not only others but also yourself. Even though your assessment reveals that you would enjoy making deep, meaningful relationships with your patients, it may be even more important for someone with your desire for connection to make sure you protect your emotional health. You will need to make sure to take time with friends and family and invest in your emotional and physical well-being. Since you are naturally wired this way, you likely have to make an extra effort *not* to take the drama home with you. Learn to leave it at the workplace, and you will have enough to give to you, your loved ones, AND your patients!

> **POWER PLAY:** Know Your Tender Spots
> Write down three patient scenarios that hit you harder than others do—and WHY.
> Was it the code on someone who was your same age? The mom who reminded you of your own?
> These aren't weaknesses. They're emotional compass points. Use them to avoid units that press too hard on old wounds—or choose to heal by walking through them with support.

Less-Emotionally Charged Departments

The OR and procedural units are generally the main departments that may be viewed as lower on the emotional yardstick. Getting to know patients and families personally is not commonly part of the daily routine of care in the OR. Nurses are focused on quick recovery and episodic patient interactions with little opportunity for emotional bonding. If you find that your personal strengths and traits are less related to emotional connections and perhaps you are more fulfilled by task completion and attention to detail, this may be a great place for you to thrive!

Remember: there's no "right" or "wrong" here. Just like some nurses love working nights, whereas others would rather quit than give up their daylight hours, it's all about finding where YOU thrive. Your emotional comfort zone is just as important as your clinical skills when it comes to job satisfaction. But finding the right fit isn't just about the work itself. It's also about how it integrates with the rest of your life. This brings us to an equally important topic: work-life balance. How do you build a career that challenges and fulfills you without sacrificing your well-being? Let's find out in the next chapter.

CHAPTER 5

Work-Life Balance

There may be no topic more important than work-life balance when it comes to choosing the right unit. Nurses who succeed at creating the right work-life balance reduce the risk of burnout prevalent among nurses who lack boundaries between the two.

In this chapter, we dig into the evidence-based reasons why work-life balance is so important and then apply the trends you uncovered for your personality traits to determine which units will best support that balance!

Terri's Testimonial

I had just badged in to work for another long shift in one of the busiest ORs in the city, preparing for the rewarding exhaustion of a 12-hour shift, when my phone buzzed. Mom. My twin sister and I were very close to our mom, but she would hardly ever call me right at the beginning of my shift. I had been working in healthcare for over 15 years, and my mother was very familiar with the routine. That said, I could always find a few minutes for the woman who so diligently had helped put me through nursing school.

I smiled, pressing the phone to my ear. "Hey, Mama. You need me to pick something up for you when I get off?"

"No, baby—my foot's been hurting. There's a sore on the bottom that won't go away. Can you stop by on your way home and take a look?"

I frowned. My mother's voice just didn't sound right. "Why didn't you say something sooner?"

"I didn't want to bother you. I know you're busy."

My heart clenched. I knew my mother meant well, but still, she should have called earlier. Diabetes wasn't something to play with.

"I'll be there around 7:45," I said, slipping the familiar OR shoe coverings over my sneakers. For the rest of the night, I was busy taking vitals, administering meds, pushing stretchers, and giving reports on my post-op patients, my mom never far from my worried mind.

As promised, I headed straight to my mother's house as soon as my shift was over. When I pulled into the driveway, something felt off. My mother was an early riser, and I could see that there was no movement in the small house—too still, too quiet.

I let myself in with my key. "Mama?"

No answer.

My pulse quickened as I moved through the house, dread settling deep in my gut.

And then I saw her.

My mother was lying on the floor by the bed, still, her skin an eerie shade of gray. I rushed to her side, shaking her.

"Mama! Wake up!"

No response. Her breathing was shallow, her pulse weak.

I grabbed my phone and dialed 911 with trembling fingers.

"I need an ambulance! My mother is unresponsive; she's diabetic, and I think she's septic."

As I waited, I checked her foot. The sore she had mentioned was black, the tissue around it mottled and swollen. Sepsis.

The EMTs arrived within minutes, though it felt like hours. I rode with them to the hospital, holding my mother's cold hand the entire way.

In the ICU, the doctors confirmed what I already knew.

"Septic shock," one of them told me gently. "It's severe. We've started broad-spectrum antibiotics, fluids, pressors...but she's not responding well."

I nodded, my sister and I holding onto each other so tightly, as if by doing so neither of us would fall. How different it felt to be on the other side of the hospital bed. As the nurse, I would have known what to do...for my patient, for the family. But this was my mother, and in this moment, I was daughter and sister, not nurse. Over the next two days, I barely left my mother's bedside. The woman who had raised me, who had worked double shifts to put me through nursing school, was now clinging to life on a ventilator.

Then came the conversation every doctor, every nurse, every loved one dreads.

"She's not improving," the doctor said, his tone gentle but firm. "At this point, we need to consider her wishes. Does she have an advance directive? What would she want?"

My throat tightened. "She never talked about it."

I turned to my sister, but her eyes were just as lost as mine.

Finally, I leaned over the bed, gripping my mother's frail hand. My voice trembled as I whispered, "Mommy, what do you want me to do?"

At that exact moment, the monitor let out a long, flat beep that sent ice through my veins.

Asystole.

I barely registered the nurse rushing in, the call for a code, the hands pushing me to the side as they started compressions.

But I knew.

My mother was gone.

I stood in the corner of the ICU room, staring blankly as the team worked, my mind echoing with that question I'd never get an answer to.

I barely remembered making the calls to family near and far. But it turned out that the most profound call wasn't to them. It was to my director at my own hospital. "I...I need some time off," I told her, my voice trembling. "My mom passed away yesterday."

There was a pause.

Then, in the most detached tone I'd ever heard, my manager said, "I'll have to check the schedule first."

My grip on the phone tightened. "Check the schedule?"

"We're already short-staffed. I can probably give you a couple of days, but a full week? I don't know."

Something inside me snapped.

"I'll be taking FMLA," I said coldly. "I'll send the paperwork." And I hung up.

When I returned to work weeks later, nothing felt the same. I couldn't separate the experiences from my mom's death from work.

Every room I walked into, every patient I saw, all blurred into the same haunting image of my mother lying in that hospital bed.

The beeping of monitors made my stomach turn. Every Code Blue made me break into a sweat.

I had believed that I was immune to the compassion fatigue and burnout I'd seen nurses go through. But I was coming to the realization that I couldn't do this anymore. Losing my mother made me realize more than ever how important family is, and I wanted to spend more time with them.

After years of working in the ICU, step-down, and PACU as a tech, LPN, and RN—from the beginning of the COVID pandemic to the end—I thought I could do that work forever. But not now. Not after what I'd been through.

The next morning, I resigned.

I didn't know where I would go next, but I knew one thing: I was at peace with leaving the bedside.

Why Work-Life Balance Matters

Work-life balance is a hot topic, and we all know it matters. So let's look at some of the research behind why it matters. In numerous studies, burnout has been shown to negatively impact patient safety, job satisfaction, and mental health.[xvii] In addition to our mental health, some studies even demonstrate that a lack of work-life balance can impact physical health. In fact, a 2019 study in the *Journal of Nursing Management* reveals that nurses working long hours or rotating shifts have a higher risk of cardiovascular disease and musculoskeletal problems.[xviii] I don't know about you, but I put in way too much effort to drink my water, exercise, and eat right only to have it all undone every shift I am at work. Furthermore, persistent stress and lack of recovery time can lead to

Nurses working long hours or rotating shifts have a higher risk of cardiovascular disease and musculoskeletal problems.

anxiety, depression, and substance use, as evidenced by research published by the Public Library of Science.[xix]

Nurse burnout and clinicians leaving the profession are a major global concern. In the United States, around 15 to 18 percent of nurses leave their jobs every year. Some hospitals even see 20 percent or more turnover annually.[xx] Reasons for this attrition range from where they're working to what their job is like and what's making them feel frustrated or over it. Studies support the notion that nurses who find a good fit within their units experience higher levels of job fulfillment and are less prone

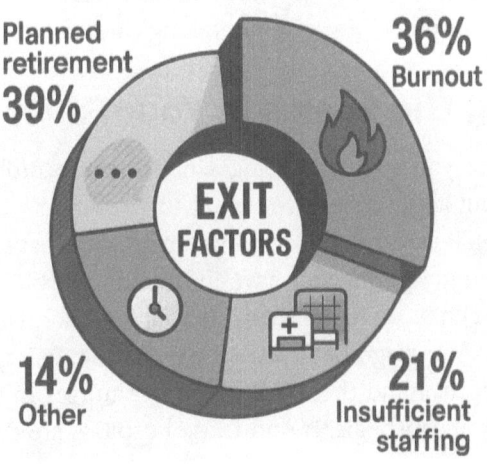

WHY NURSES LEAVE THE PROFESSION

- Planned retirement 39%
- Burnout 36%
- Insufficient staffing 21%
- Other 14%

EXIT FACTORS

to burnout.[xxi] This is what we are talking about here. If we can help reduce this inherent stress by being in a department that is the right fit for our individual personalities and strengths, then shouldn't we do it?

Nursing is a physically demanding, emotionally exhausting profession. Additionally, common expectations such as required night or weekend shifts and working holidays represent likely intrusions into personal time for adequate sleep, self-care, and time with friends and loved ones. There is also a growing trend toward mandatory overtime in many hospitals to combat short staffing due to widespread nursing shortages. But even voluntary overtime can be a real threat to work-life balance. When your supervisor calls you up offering all sorts of incentives such as paying you at time and a half or pleads with you about how much the unit needs you, it's hard to say no. I am no stranger to picking up more work because I felt bad about leaving the unit short-staffed. As a new nurse, I remember thinking that it would win me favor with my leaders and coworkers if I picked up extra shifts here and there. Truth be told, I think it was more harmful to my well-being than it was helpful to the unit and the patients.

We owe it to ourselves, our friends and families, and, yes, our patients to take care of ourselves. What shape will you be in to take care of others if you're not taking care of yourself?

Tipping the Scales in Your Favor

Since before you started nursing school, you've probably been daydreaming about where you want to work and what kind of patients you'll care for. But what you might not have realized is just how many options you have in nursing. Beyond the different departments, there are many specialties, each with its own unique mix of diagnoses, procedures, and nursing considerations. Keep in mind that 63.2 percent of nurses in the United States work in hospitals.[xxii] And those hospitals are divided into departments based on specialties; there is no "one size fits all" in nursing. However, nursing-school curriculums are generic and exist to give you a solid foundation to pass NCLEX for licensure.

The wonderful education you've received is only the beginning. You will get the specific training you need after you are hired and complete hospital and unit orientation. Depending on the type of nursing program you attend—two-year associate's, four-year bachelor's, accelerated bachelor's—after a year of nursing residency, you will have invested at least three years of education and training to become a fully functioning nurse in your department. You and your personal well-being are worth the brief time it will take to make sure that you choose the optimal unit.

Make no mistake: no matter where you work in the hospital setting, you will have to be very intentional about maintaining a work-life balance. Selecting a unit that complements your strengths can significantly enhance job satisfaction. Hospital shifts are long in the OR and in the inpatient units. Some departments and hospitals offer shorter shifts, but keep in mind that they are the exception and not the rule. As you start your journey transitioning from nursing student to professional nurse, make sure you plan for your own well-being and self-care, feeling empowered that when it comes to achieving work-life balance, you are looking after your mental health, maximizing resilience, and protecting the investment you've made in yourself!

A Real Balancing Act

As I mentioned at the very beginning of this book, nursing is tough, but it is also very rewarding. Big picture: the key to work-life balance is making sure the tough parts don't outweigh the rewarding parts. Ideally, it's the opposite and the rewarding part outweighs the tough part. That's how we achieve job satisfaction, provide excellent care, and stay in the profession for the long term.

Now let's discuss specific personality traits and how they can support work-life balance in different units. Do you tend to take great pride in having a strong work ethic? Pay close attention to what is being asked here! This is not a question of your *willingness* or *ability* to work hard. The question is whether high productivity and task completion make you feel fulfilled. If so, you are probably at a high risk for burnout due to a lack of work-life balance. You are more likely to pick up the extra shifts, skip lunch breaks, and work longer hours. And all this is more likely to occur in the ICU, ER, and OR.

In the ICU and ER, admissions are unpredictable, which can mean nurses may have to work longer hours during their shift. For instance, I can recall working in the burn ICU and staying over six hours after the end of my shift, which was the longest I'd ever stayed over. Fifteen minutes before the end of my shift, a mom and her two toddlers were admitted for significant burns and smoke inhalation from a house fire. It was one of those "all hands on deck" situations that would surely make you feel guilty about clocking out and heading home.

Every nurse will, at some point, find themselves in the same predicament: exhausted and stressed out after a long 12-hour shift but faced with the choice of whether to keep going. Though a lack of work-life balance can happen in every department, there is simply a greater risk in the ED and ICU, where high acuity levels often make it difficult to transfer care to the next caregiver just because the clock hits 7:00. Likewise, in the OR, complicated surgeries can extend beyond the end of a shift or into a lunch break, making it difficult for an OR nurse to leave the surgical suite.

In addition to your passion for hard work (or lack thereof), another personality trait to consider when choosing your unit is your need to direct or be in control. People with these personality types struggle with delegation, which is a key strategy in managing stress in departments that are extremely task heavy.

Work-Life Balance

In departments such as the ICU, ER, and OR, the need to be in control is, for the most part, an asset, but it needs to be balanced with delegation to prevent stress and burnout from overcommitment. In other words, control what you must control and delegate the rest whenever you start to feel overwhelmed.

Departments like med-surg and oncology are not immune to threats to work-life balance. Though it's not ideal, med-surg nurses can routinely have five to six patients a shift (unless you practice in a state with strict nurse-patient ratios, which we will talk about later). The reason these departments may be slightly less impactful in terms of work-life balance is that the patients are generally less critically ill. For instance, the chances of having a patient code with a long resuscitation that has you on your feet for extended periods of time that go into your lunch break or extend past the end of your shift are far greater in the ICU and ED than in other departments.

> **POWER PLAY:** Schedule Joy Like a Shift
> This week, put one joy-filled activity on your calendar with the same respect as you would a work shift.
> Make sure you don't cancel it. Don't "reschedule" it into oblivion.
> Balance isn't what you squeeze in. It's what you protect.
> Balance doesn't happen after burnout. It happens in the margins of every week.

Let's consider this question again. Do high productivity and task completion make you feel fulfilled? If the answer is no, why risk burnout in a department that does not check that box for you? Remember: one of the top-three causes of burnout and why nurses leave the profession is work-life balance, so this is a critical consideration when you are choosing a unit.

Think honestly about how you are fulfilled from your work productivity so you can balance the scales in your favor;

work-life balance is key, but it's not the only unit characteristic to consider. Furthermore, there may be other personality traits that still make the ED, OR, or ICU a good fit for you, like it is for many others. One major factor? Autonomy. The ability to make decisions, act, and use your clinical judgment without constant oversight can make all the difference in job satisfaction. So just like we would with our patients, let's keep going with our head-to-toe assessment and explore the role of autonomy in shaping your nursing career.

CHAPTER 6

You've Got the Power

Autonomy in nursing is all about making your own clinical decisions within your scope of practice. It means using your judgment, skills, and training to act without waiting for constant direction. Autonomy exists on a spectrum, and your preference often connects to your personality traits such as confidence, risk tolerance, desire for structure, and communication style.[xxiii]

In this chapter, we review different units with high and moderate levels of autonomy, then consider how you might fit in various units based on your personality and how important it is for you to have independence when making clinical decisions.

Nina's Narrative

Med-surg—I felt like I had finally made it. I just knew I was about to change the world! I had dreamed of the moment when I would have my first patient assignments: fresh scrubs on, stethoscope around my neck, ready to rock and roll! I welcomed the steady beeping of monitors, the hum of conversation at the nurses' station, the feeling of purpose. I was finally a nurse, and that meant everything to me.

And for a while, that was enough. In fact, it was more than enough. I thrived on the variety, the way no two shifts were ever the same. I liked that I never knew whether I'd be handling post-op recoveries, chronic illness management, or an unexpected rapid response. There was always something new to figure out, always a problem to solve. I was constantly learning and growing.

But over time, something shifted. It was gradual, like water wearing down a stone. It happened in moments subtle at first, then undeniably grew like a snowball—and not the soft, fluffy kind but like the ones full of cold ice that sting when you get hit by one.

There was that shift when I had to take care of 13 patients. Thirteen! The number sat heavily in my brain as I counted the names on my list, hoping I had made a mistake and that I was not about to put my license at risk with so many patients. I had barely introduced myself to my last patient when my first one was already overdue for meds. I told my charge nurse that I was concerned about patient safety. I would look down the hallway to see the glow of call lights over my patient rooms that never seemed to go away, a visible reminder of my inability to keep up. I moved from room to room, answering questions, assessing vitals, passing medications, abandoning the hope of documenting anything. At a certain point, my back and legs ached so much that I felt like I had been treading water for hours. There was no pause, no breath—just a constant, desperate attempt not to miss something important. By the end of my shift, I wasn't sure if I had really helped anyone at all. In that moment, I felt as though I had no control over my own nursing practice.

Then there was the night of the unassigned patient. I remember hearing the overhead pages on the intercom: "Patient needs nurse assistance in room 31. Patient needs assistance in room 31." Her voice had a sharp edge, a note of urgency that cut through the usual background noise of the floor. I kept thinking, "Where is that patient's nurse?" After four hours into the shift, I stopped at the nurses' station and asked if the nurse for room 31 was stuck in another patient's room and needed help. The charge nurse looked at the assignment sheet and suddenly realized that she'd never assigned a nurse to the patient! And of course, I got to be the lucky nurse who would now have to walk into this patient's room. My chest tightened as I imagined the quiet panic this patient likely felt, pressing the call button, *watching the door, waiting for someone who wasn't coming. It would have been a rough night for him to say the least.*

And then there was the thyroidectomy patient. The one who couldn't breathe.

I knew something was wrong the moment I walked in. There's a certain way panic looks in a patient's eyes—wider, wilder, desperate for someone to do something. His breaths were shallow, his fingers twitching toward his throat, trying to explain what his body wouldn't let him say. I called the provider. No answer. I called again.

"He's fine," one of the other nurses told me. "It's just post-op swelling."

But something inside me screamed, "No, it's not!"

I tried again.

"I think we need to do something," I urged.

I was met with sighs and dismissive glances. I was being dramatic. Overreacting. I doubted myself in that moment, thinking maybe I was imagining it, maybe I was too green, too eager to sound the alarm.

I felt powerless to help this patient until the nurse manager passed by the room and I convinced her to come in and take a look. Her eyes grew wide as she quickly assessed the patient and realized that he was in trouble. She immediately called the attending physician and had the patient transferred to the ICU. I was right.

It took a long time for me to stop hearing the echoes of that shift in my head. The way I had spoken up but been ignored. The way I had known something was wrong but had felt powerless to act.

But I wasn't powerless, I realized much later. I just hadn't found the right way to use my voice.

The work was important. I knew that. But I started to feel like a passenger instead of the driver. I was moving, reacting, responding, but was I in control?

After three years, I wasn't sure how much more I had to give. Not to the patients—I always had something left for them—but to the way things worked and the constant battle to feel like I had a say in what happened next. I was ready to get away, get out, and leave nursing.

Then, I learned that the OR was hiring, so I transferred to that unit. It was easy; the OR had gone through a mass exodus after the department leader retired. My med-surg skills were super transferable, and they were simply looking for experienced nurses.

I wasn't sure what drew me to it. Maybe it was curiosity. Maybe it was the need for something different. Maybe I just wanted to feel in control again.

The first time I stepped into the OR, it felt like walking into another world. Everything was intentional, structured. There was no chaos, no alarms ringing in the distance, no scramble to keep up with a patient load too heavy to carry. The OR wasn't about keeping up. It was about leading.

I was no longer bouncing from room to room, pulled in a dozen directions at once. In the OR, I had one patient. One focus. One responsibility. And in that space, I had a level of autonomy I hadn't realized I was missing.

As a circulating nurse, I orchestrated the room and thrived in this culture built on the unspoken communication between the team, the anticipation of what was needed before it was asked for, the constant awareness of everything happening at once. If something was wrong, I didn't wait for someone else to notice. If a patient wasn't positioned correctly, if a protocol wasn't being followed, if sterility was compromised, I spoke up, and people listened.

There were no distractions, no overflowing assignment lists, no moments of hesitation when I wondered whether I should push harder for what I knew was right. The OR gave me space to trust my instincts, to act with confidence, to take ownership of a patient's safety in a way I had never been able to before.

Sure, I missed the long conversations with patients, the moments of connection with families, the way I could see someone's progress over days in med-surg. But in the OR, I found something else: clarity, control, and the power to make sure that my patient, that one single person on the table, was protected.

In med-surg, I had been part of the bigger picture, a vital thread in a massive web of care. In the OR, I was the guardian standing at the door.

I had found my place. I had found my voice.

And I would never give that up again.

Shot Caller

Okay, so it might be a slight exaggeration to say that nurses "call the shots" (not really, just keeping the scope-of-practice police at bay!). In any case, as discussed, there are certain departments in a hospital where nurses exercise a greater amount of autonomy than they do in others. Patient conditions in the ICU and ED can change in an instant. In the OR, where nurses also exercise a great deal of autonomy, the nurse is usually the coordinator of the entire room, ensuring patient safety by maintaining sterility, visually assessing the patient, and basically keeping an eye on everything going on in the surgical suite. There isn't always time to wait, and nurses must make decisions in seconds, with little to no input, to save a patient's life and maintain patient safety.

For you, one of these departments may sound like the perfect place. Your patient's stable blood pressure suddenly drops. You will likely need to titrate up on the Levophed. Then you walk in the room to find your patient agitated and breathing over the ventilator. Will you titrate the fentanyl or the Ativan? You will likely make the decision based on your clinical judgment. You walk into the surgical suite and notice that a patient who is under conscious sedation is turning purple. You inform the anesthetist and surgeon that intubation may be necessary.

If you're the type of person who enjoys taking charge, thinking critically under pressure, and making judgment calls with confidence, a high-autonomy department might be your best fit. If your personality assessment shows that you are assertive, decisive, and persuasive, you would likely feel right at home.

Not every nurse wants or needs that level of autonomy to feel fulfilled. Many nurses prefer a balance of independence and structured support, where they still have a say in patient care but within a team-driven, collaborative environment. Independent decision-making exists but in a less high-acuity setting. Medical-surgical, labor and delivery, behavioral health, and oncology offer that mix, allowing nurses to make important decisions while following structured protocols and collaborating closely with providers. These nurses thrive in a setting where teamwork is central, routines provide stability, and communication is key.

Impact on Job Satisfaction

If you're a new nurse, autonomy can make or break your job satisfaction. Having to think on your feet, handle challenges, and make decisions on your own (within your scope of practice, of course!) can help you feel more in control and less overwhelmed. The right unit can push you to grow while still giving you the support you need. Plus, nurses with more autonomy can step in faster when something goes wrong, improving patient care and outcomes.

On the flip side, the expectation that you may have to make critical clinical decisions may not appeal to you. You may not be comfortable with that role or see no added value in enduring more required education, more certifications, and longer department orientations. Additionally, you will be required to have a firm handle on the policies and protocols that keep you within your nursing scope of practice. For example, titrated medications such as Levophed or Precedex keep patients alive, but incorrect titration can lead to death. There is rarely a physician standing by to inform the ICU nurse that it's time to titrate. Titration orders will include the parameters for titration based on clinical condition, vital signs, and responses to any number of interventions. It is the nurse's responsibility to decide the appropriate interventions based on the data reflecting the patient's condition.

As a burn-ICU nurse, I had to have BLS, ACLS, ABLS, and PALS certifications. I recall how one of my good friends from nursing school, Merita, a brilliant med-surg nurse, jokingly asked me, "Honey, why would you want to work there? I only have my BLS; I follow my orders and escalate when I need to. Plus, you and I get paid the same hourly rate."

Now, Merita was playing down the level of autonomy in med-surg (there is quite a bit). In any case, she sure had a point, but I found that level of autonomy thrilling. Why? Because I had a different personality and different strengths than she did.

"Different strokes for different folks, I guess," I replied.

Not every unit will be the right fit for your level of comfort with autonomy or your desire to have it, and that's okay. If you love high-pressure environments, you might thrive in the ER, where you're expected to act fast and make judgment calls before the medical provider can arrive. If you're more into critical thinking with close monitoring and data-informed decision-making, the ICU could be your place. Behavioral-health nurses also have a lot of independence when it comes to de-escalating crises and implementing patient-care plans. Finding a unit that matches your confidence level and gives you room to grow will help you feel more in control of your career and set you up for success.

Nurse autonomy is everywhere in the hospital, but how much say-so you have depends on the unit. Some areas call for quick, independent decision-making, whereas others are more team driven with set protocols. Either way, nursing expertise is an integral part of the care plan.

Keep in mind, though, that the level of autonomy may also be influenced by the type of hospital and how protocols are utilized by the facility. These characterizations are representative of how most (but not all) departments function.

> **POWER PLAY:** Flip the Scene; Find Your Voice
> Think back to a moment during clinicals orientation, or a shift where you weren't the decision-maker.
>
> Maybe your preceptor took over.
> Maybe the doctor made a choice that you didn't understand.
> Maybe you froze and stayed quiet when you wanted to speak up.
>
> Now, grab your journal or notes app and answer this question:
>
> *If you had full autonomy in that moment, what would you have done differently?*
> *What would you have said, asked, or done?*
> *How would you have felt before, during, and after?*
>
> This is not about *right or wrong*. This is about clarity. Ownership. **Truth.**

Guided Independence

Which level of autonomy sounds like you? Do you thrive when making fast decisions with little oversight, or do you prefer a role where guidelines and collaboration help shape patient care? Neither path is necessarily better than the other. It's all about finding the right fit for you. The best way to feel confident and fulfilled as a nurse is to match your strengths to an environment that makes you feel empowered, whether that means working independently in a fast-paced unit or thriving in a setting where teamwork and structure provide the foundation.

No matter where you work, one thing remains true: nurses play a critical role in patient care, and autonomy exists in every setting. The key is finding a unit where the level of independence and control feels just right, because when you're in the right place, you don't just survive as a nurse. You thrive.

And as nursing continues to evolve, so does the technology that supports it. From electronic health records to AI-assisted diagnostics, innovation is transforming the way nurses deliver care. In the next chapter, we explore how technology is shaping the future of nursing and how you can use it to enhance both efficiency and patient outcomes.

CHAPTER 7

Tech It or Leave It

Nursing is no longer just about hands-on care. It's also about knowing how to navigate the technology that keeps patients safe and (fingers crossed) makes your job a little easier. But how much is too much…for you, that is? This chapter is going to help you figure that out. We break down how different units use technology so you can find your fit and be confident stepping into whatever environment feels right for you. We start with comparing units where technology is deeply embedded in the daily workflow versus those that may use less and then identify your personality traits that align with each setting. Let's go!

Darby's Depiction

The ICU is not for the faint of heart. Some days, it feels like you don't even have time to breathe. Six months in, I had learned to weather the storm of beeping monitors, rapid-fire assessments, and split-second decisions that could mean the difference between life and death.

All through nursing school, this was my dream unit. But, if I were being honest, I started having doubts about my choice since I'd been working there. I had even begun to wonder if nursing was the right fit for me. Cue the dramatic life crisis.

I still remember the moment when I hit my breaking point. It was toward the end of a brutal shift, just one more hour before I could clock out and face plant into my bed. I was in a patient's room, trying to wrap up some documentation (because what's nursing without endless charting, right?). Then it happened. The ventilator alarm started blaring out of nowhere. EEEEE. EEEEE. EEEEE. It was the low-pressure alarm.

I spun around, my heart pounding. My patient, a 64-year-old post-cardiac-arrest survivor, wasn't looking so good. His oxygen levels were dropping fast. His chest? Barely moving. The vent wasn't pushing air into his lungs.

My first thought was, "Okay, stay calm; this is fine." My second thought? "Shoot, I don't know what the hell I'm doing!"

I checked the tubing. No kinks, no obstructions, and the ET tube was connected, as far as I could tell. My heart was racing as I started pressing buttons on the vent like I was trying to reboot an old laptop. I know, I know—you're not supposed to mess with the settings, but where was respiratory? Where was anyone?!

This was a brand-new ventilator, a fancy upgrade, courtesy of the hospital. I thought I had learned the basics during the training from the vendor, but suddenly all that knowledge flew right out of my head.

Cue internal panic. Cue beads of sweat on my forehead like I was in a nursing version of *Who Wants to Be a Millionaire?* and had just used my last lifeline.

The nurse from the room next door rushed in, and without thinking, I asked him to disconnect my patient from the vent and start bagging while I called respiratory, who said that they were on the way. I turned back to the ventilator, desperately trying to override the alarm, looking lost and confused.

EEEEE, EEEEE, EEEEE. Push this button. Error.

EEEEE, EEEEE, EEEEE. Press that button. Error.

The numbers on the screen started to blur. My breath felt tight; my hands were shaky. Was this stress? A panic attack? Or was I just not cut out for this?

The attending finally showed up, eyes darting from the patient to the vent. "What's happening?"

I swallowed hard. "The vent isn't cycling right; I can't clear the alarm."

"Try putting it in standby and resetting it," he suggested.

I nodded, fumbling with the buttons like it was my first time trying to operate a ventilator. Beep. Error. Fantastic.

That's when Yvette, one of the senior nurses, swooped in, cool as ever. She pressed a combo of buttons like she had a secret cheat code, and just like that, the vent reset. Magic. We reconnected my patient, and slowly—thankfully!—his chest started rising again. I let out a breath I hadn't even realized I was holding in.

Yvette gave my shoulder a squeeze. "Hey, you're not alone. We're all still figuring out these machines." I managed a weak laugh. But inside? I was spiraling. The truth hit me hard: I wasn't learning; I was drowning.

This wasn't just about one vent malfunction or one chaotic shift. It was every shift. The endless documentation. The constant fear of missing something. At the end of most of my shifts, even though I was helping the sickest of patients, I was not fulfilled, only frustrated.

That night, I faced what I had been too scared to admit. I couldn't do this anymore. I was so done with spending more time with ventilators, medication pumps, and CRRT machines than I did with actual patients. I didn't want to feel like I was drowning in numbers, alarms, and tech anymore. I wanted to be on a floor where I could truly connect with my patients, where I could breathe.

By the end of that shift, I knew. It wasn't that I didn't love nursing. I did. But I needed a different kind of challenge and a different kind of intensity. Something that didn't leave me feeling empty and drained by the time I walked out those double doors at the end of the day.

So I made the call: I was leaving the ICU.

And let me tell you, that decision didn't feel like quitting. It felt like I was choosing me.

A month later, I transferred to oncology. It wasn't long before I realized I had found my place. Sure, machines were still there, but the focus? It was on building relationships with my patients, supporting them and getting to know their stories.

That was five years ago, and I've never looked back.

Tech-Intensive Units: For the Detail Oriented, Analytical, and Focused

Let's get to it. Some nursing units are straight-up tech heavy. These units generally include the ICU and ED, where machines are constantly buzzing, monitors are flashing numbers at you, and your brain has to stay sharp 24/7. Because you're caring for the sickest patients in these departments, you will be surrounded by some of the most advanced equipment in the hospital, which require frequent changes and updates so that these high-acuity patients receive the most innovative and advanced care possible.

Are you the type of person who thrives on solving complex problems and isn't scared of data overload? You might be built for these high-tech environments. If you love the idea of working with ventilators, smart infusion pumps, and real-time patient monitoring, you might thrive in a tech-heavy environment.

If you are analytical and deliberate, you might find the use of technology and applying data from monitors and machines a great addition to your bedside care. As a matter of fact, you will likely love having the objective data measurements to help you know what is going on with your patients. Additionally, those who love the challenge of learning how to use new tools and equipment thrive in these settings. If you're someone who loves a challenge, thrives on details, and has laser-sharp focus, this could be your playground. While you're juggling complex tech setups, you will need to be cool as a cucumber to handle life-or-death decisions. If you love solving puzzles and find satisfaction in precision, you'll feel right at home there. You will also need to have a love for learning.

When evaluating your assessment results, those who show personality traits that are more aligned with introverted work and comfortable with making decisions based on instinct would likely thrive in this environment where the strategic, process-oriented workflows engage those natural tendencies. On the other hand, if you take the OCEAN assessment and score high in agreeableness, you may thrive on human connection, which can sometimes take a backseat in tech-heavy departments.

Less Tech-Intensive Units: For the Organized and Compassionate

Whereas some nursing units are tech heavy, others are not quite as reliant on machines (although such equipment is always important). In departments such as med-surg, oncology, and L&D, you'll still use technology daily, but it won't completely run the show. You'll get a good mix of hands-on care and tech-driven tasks, perfect for those who want some balance.

If you want to ensure that you will spend more time with patients than with machines, you may find that these departments are the right space for you. You're not all about being surrounded by blinking machines 24/7. You still want to work with tech, but you want to ensure that you have a solid patient interaction. That's where these units shine.

Take, for example, Michael, a new nurse starting his shift on a busy med-surg floor. First thing? He pulls up his patient list in the hospital's EHR, prioritizing who needs attention first. His first patient has scheduled meds, so he grabs the BCMA scanner and double-checks everything because one missed detail could mean a med error, and he's not about that life.

Midway through the shift, a smart bed alarm goes off—someone's trying to get up on their own. Michael jumps in, checks their vitals using the bedside monitor, and makes sure that they're safe before moving on. Later, he catches an irregular heart rate on a telemetry read, calls the NP, and helps catch a potential complication before it escalates.

Michael's superpower? He's organized, thorough, and compassionate. He knows how to use tech to his advantage without letting it pull him away from patient care.

Let's look at the OCEAN assessment as another example. A score that places you smack dab in the middle of the spectrum for openness would indicate that you are open to incorporating new technology into your daily workflow. You're not excited about the new high-tech monitors. You're also not banging your head against your locker because they will throw off your whole routine. If that sounds like you, tech savvy but also patient focused, these units could be where you'd thrive.

Least Tech-Intensive Unit: For the Therapist at Heart

Behavioral health is the unit that uses the least amount of technology because the outcomes associated with the diagnoses are not measured by a piece of equipment. Rather, it's all about *behavior*, with a focus on emotional connection, communication, and supporting patients through some of life's toughest moments. In behavioral health, technology takes a back seat. You'll use EHRs for documentation and basic physical monitoring, but the real work happens through therapeutic conversations and emotional support. It's all about building trust, listening, and helping patients through mental-health challenges.

This space is not for everyone. If you're someone who is very detail oriented and precise, you might find the slower pace and lack of measurable outcomes frustrating. On the other hand, let's say you took the OCEAN assessment and you scored high in openness to experiences. You may be more comfortable in behavioral health, where you navigate more ambiguous situations such as responding to a patient's unpredictable mood swings without relying on an alarm or lab result to guide you.

Like It or Not, Technology Is Here to Stay

Not to age myself, but I still remember when paper charting was a thing. I recall the ease of flipping through my flowsheet or my MAR and quickly finding whatever information I needed in the chart. It was a real change when everything went into the computer. Thankfully, I was a fairly new nurse when we made the transition to the EMR and did not have the same challenges as some of the more experienced nursing colleagues who charted on paper for many years. I remember our manager warning us: "Well, you all better get used to it. This is just the beginning!"

Looking back, she totally nailed it. Artificial intelligence, predictive analytics, and wearable health technology are changing the game. Technology isn't coming. It's already here, boots on the ground. AI is showing up in hospitals in some wild ways, from employing virtual sitters to help prevent falls to scanning diagnostic images faster than we could ever pull them up on the screen. Predictive analytics? That's your behind-the-scenes teammate flagging early signs of sepsis or heart failure before the vitals tank.

Wearable tech such as wireless bio-patch sensors and continuous glucose monitors are becoming standard issue, especially in such units as the ICU and ED, where real-time data can be the difference between stabilizing a patient or calling a code. Whether it's scanning meds, watching vitals tick in real time, or robotic-assisted surgeries that look straight out of a sci-fi movie, tech is touching every corner of care.

Some units are already deep in the game, fully wired and teched out. Others are easing in. But the truth is that no matter what unit you're in, the future of nursing isn't tech *versus* touch. It's learning to weave them together.

> **POWER PLAY:** Try the Tech-Free Test
> Plan a One-Shift Challenge: Notice how you feel during tasks that don't require tech.
>
> Example: emotional support, wound care, feeding, repositioning, basic hygiene.
>
> Do you feel more present? More fulfilled? Or kind of bored?
>
> This isn't about judgment—it's about joy.

Find Your Zone and Own It

As is surely very apparent by now, nursing doesn't look the same for everyone. What is also very apparent by now (at least I hope!) is that that's the beauty of it! Some nurses thrive when surrounded by high-tech machines and critical decisions. Others shine brightest in quieter spaces where the focus is on deep, meaningful connection and prefer not to have to focus on using high-tech equipment.

The key is knowing yourself. Are you all about that tech-driven environment where every beep matters? Or do you need room for connection, reflection, and conversation without the constant buzz of machines?

Wherever your strengths lie, there's a unit out there that's going to feel like home. Trust your instincts, lean into what excites you, and don't be afraid to push yourself. You have the skills. You just need the right space to let them shine. In the next chapter, we dive deeper into the wide variety of units in a hospital, from high-intensity trauma centers to quieter specialty floors, so you can find the environment where you'll not only thrive but also truly love what you do.

CHAPTER 8

Variety

One of the best things about nursing is that no two shifts are ever the same. Depending on where you work, you might be starting IVs on a trauma patient, admitting a first-time mom in labor, stabilizing someone in septic shock, or de-escalating a psych crisis, all in one shift. The variety of diagnoses you'll see depends on the unit, and that variety can shape your skills, confidence, and overall job satisfaction.

Some nurses love the adrenaline rush of the ER, where every patient experience brings something completely different. Others prefer the controlled chaos of the ICU, where even though the diagnoses are critical, they're often similar, allowing for deeper expertise. And then there are nurses who thrive in med-surg or oncology, managing a steady mix of chronic and acute conditions. Whatever your style, knowing how much variety you'll see in each specialty can help you figure out where you'll fit best.

In this chapter, we explore the amount of variety you may see throughout the hospital. From the wide range of conditions in the emergency department to the more focused, specialized care in L&D, every unit tells a different clinical story. If you're still exploring where you belong, understanding what kinds of cases show up on each floor can help you choose a unit that aligns with how your brain works and what excites you clinically. Let's break it down because the more you know about the variety in each unit, the easier it'll be to find the one that fits you.

Marcus's Moment

I glanced at the whiteboard as I walked into the unit around 6:45 a.m., coffee in hand and stethoscope draped around my neck, ready to start the day. The charge nurse had already given me a heads-up that I'd be getting the first post-op admission later in the day and was starting with three patients, none of them with the same diagnosis. That made me smile.

This is exactly why I chose med-surg.

Some of my friends in the ICU and ER keep me entertained with wild stories about crashing patients and adrenaline-packed moments. But me? I found my rhythm in the organized chaos of med-surg. It's not simple, and that's what continues to draw me to it. Each shift throws something new at me. One moment, I'm managing antibiotics; the next, I'm de-escalating a confused patient or stabilizing someone fresh from the ICU. I like the rhythm. I like the unpredictability. And I'm proud of how fast I've learned to think on my feet.

I took a few minutes to go through my patients' charts and started jotting down my "brain": a folded piece of paper I keep in my pocket with the most important care details. I lucked out and found a fully charged WOW (workstation on wheels) parked right by my first patient's room. I smiled. "It's going to be a great day."

7:08 a.m., room 420. Mr. Kay, 78 years old, recovering from left hip surgery. On paper, this looked like a typical post-op, day-two case: manage pain, assist with mobility, get him up for PT. But as I helped him out of bed for a linen change, he winced and said, "I just don't feel like myself today."

I checked in with the tech for his latest vitals. Temp was up. He was more disoriented than I remembered from yesterday's shift.

Already running through the possibilities in my head, I called the physician. "I hope he's not septic." The doc gave a verbal order for fluids and a blood culture. I put in the orders and hung the fluids.

There was no time to waste; you don't stay in one room for long in med-surg.

Next stop: 422B. Layla, 24, admitted overnight for a sickle-cell crisis.

She barely looked up when I entered. She was curled in on herself, clearly in pain, her PCA pump blinking quietly. I adjusted her pillows, did a quick head-to-toe, and confirmed her pump settings.

"It's like my bones are burning," she whispered.

I nodded. My uncle has sickle-cell disease, and I've seen this pain up close. I gently refit her nasal cannula, which had slipped off, and secured the tubing behind her ears.

"Let's see how the PCA works for you," I said as I dimmed the lights and pulled the blinds closed. "If the pain doesn't start to let up, I'll call the doctor."

She gave a small nod as I slipped out.

Room 415. Mr. Rodriguez was having a rough morning.

His pneumonia had settled right on top of his COPD. When I walked in, he was clearly struggling with his BiPAP mask, clawing at it, anxious, restless. The night nurse had mentioned that he'd kept removing it overnight.

I sat down beside him and gently placed my hand on the bed rail. "Let's take a breath together," I said. "In for two...and out for three."

Once his breathing slowed, I adjusted the mask for a better seal and called the respiratory therapist. "He may need a bronchodilator," I suggested before finishing his assessment and reinforcing the importance of his keeping the mask on.

On my way back down the hall, I peeked in on Layla. She looked a little more relaxed. The morphine was doing its thing.

Then back to Mr. Kay, who was now getting a blood culture drawn by the phlebotomist.

I helped my patients with breakfast, gave meds, and made it to the morning safety huddle. Just as I reached for my now cold coffee and considered getting some documentation done, the charge nurse came around the corner.

> "Hey, Marcus, your admit is on his way—68-year-old post-op adrenalectomy, history of early onset dementia. OR just finished."
>
> 11:47 a.m. Of course. And I had never taken care of a patient after an adrenalectomy.
>
> I knew if I didn't grab lunch now, I might not eat at all. I scarfed down a sandwich in the breakroom in record time and made it back just in time to receive my new patient.
>
> By 7:15 p.m., I was giving my report. My calves were tight, my back ached, and I had a mystery stain on my scrub top. But honestly? I felt good.
>
> Four patients. Four completely different diagnoses. One post-op admit I'd never had before.
>
> It wasn't a flashy day. No codes. No traumas. But I had managed four very different patients, adapted to every challenge, and gave good care.
>
> That's why I'm here.
>
> Med-surg isn't glamorous. It's not always dramatic. But it's where I get to grow, learn, and make a real difference every single shift. And for me? That's more than enough.

Variety Is the Spice of Life—or So They Say

Some 18th-century poet once declared that "variety is the spice of life." Cool. But let's be real—some folks can handle a full spice rack, whereas others start sweating over a dash of black pepper. Case in point: my husband, born and raised in Jamaica, thinks my spice tolerance is downright tragic. Every time I try to eat jerk chicken, I have a tall glass of ice water on standby like I'm about to run a marathon, except the only thing running is my nose! Meanwhile, he's over there, casually enjoying his plate like it's mashed potatoes. Clearly, when it comes to how much spice or variety, people enjoy varying degrees. Get it? *Degrees*...heat... spice. Okay, so back to variety in a hospital...

The Variety Spectrum: Which Units Keep Things Interesting?

It's important to consider the different types of diagnoses you might manage in your department and whether the idea of more or less is appealing to you. If you like the idea of never knowing what's coming through the door next, certain nursing units will bring more excitement than others will. On the flip side, if you prefer more routine and predictability, there are units for that too. Let's break it down.

ED

By far, the department that sees the largest variety is the ED. On average, 70 percent of patients admitted to the hospital come through the ED. Imagine: that's 70 percent of all the broken bones, heart attacks, strokes, imminent births, mental breakdowns, gunshot wounds, and every other conceivable medical emergency passing through the emergency department. Whew! If you want to see it all, the ED is the place to be. Many patients who come through the ED don't get admitted to the hospital. As one of my ED friends put it, "Sometimes we just treat 'em and street 'em!"—a blunt but honest way of saying that many patients just need to be stabilized before heading home or following up outpatient with a primary provider or specialist.

Med-Surg: The Ultimate "Jack of All Trades" Unit

If you want to see a little bit of everything, med-surg is your best bet. One shift, you're taking care of a post-op appendectomy patient, someone in DKA, a patient recovering from pneumonia, and someone with chronic heart failure who came in for fluid overload. It's like a nursing variety pack: you might get a mix of wound care, pain management, telemetry monitoring, and a little bit of everything else.

That said, not all med-surg floors are created equal. Some hospitals have specialized med-surg units, such as ortho, neuro, or cardiac, where you'll see mostly the same conditions repeatedly. This makes them feel a bit more structured but also gives you exposure to a lot of different patient-care skills.

ICU: High Acuity, Same Core Focus

ICUs can also be general or specialized, just like med-surg. Some hospitals have one big medical ICU (MICU) that takes in any critically ill patient, whereas others break it down into cardiac ICU, trauma ICU, neuro ICU, etc.

But here's the difference: ICU nursing is less about variety in diagnoses and more about managing the critical aspects of care. No matter what brought a patient into the ICU, you'll likely be dealing with ventilators, sedation, titrated drips, and the constant monitoring of vital signs. So though the reasons people end up in the ICU vary, the day-to-day work of an ICU nurse stays consistent.

Behavioral Health: Different Diagnoses, Similar Care Plans

Psych nursing sits in the middle of the variety spectrum. Though behavioral-health nurses see a mix of conditions such as schizophrenia, bipolar disorder, and major depression, the overall care approach tends to focus on stabilization, medication compliance, and emotional support. So though the patient stories and interactions are different, the nursing care follows a familiar rhythm.

Labor and Delivery: Predictable but High Stakes

L&D might be one of the most routine inpatient departments, simply because the patient population is limited. After all, only half the population can have a baby! Most hospitals even split women's health into separate units:

Variety

- L&D—focuses on labor and birth
- Mother/Baby—handles postpartum care after delivery

Even within high-risk pregnancies, the daily work in L&D stays structured: fetal monitoring, pain management, coaching moms through labor, and assisting in deliveries.

The OR: High Variety, Repetitive Role

Here's the plot twist: The operating room sees the widest variety of patients, in every condition, every age, every level of severity. But for the nurses, the daily tasks don't change much. Whether you're a circulating nurse (managing the OR team and patient safety) or a scrub nurse (assisting the surgeon directly), your role is structured.

POWER PLAY Mini Quiz: "Do You Thrive with Variety or Just Survive It?"
Find out how much variety works for you in a nursing unit.

Personality Quiz

https://auspicious-water-67783.myflodesk.com/quiz

Personality Traits and the Variety Spectrum in Nursing

As discussed, different nursing units demand different levels of adaptability, learning, and variety. Your personality plays a huge role in how well you thrive in each environment. Some nurses crave constant change, whereas others prefer predictability. Here's how different traits align along the variety spectrum:

In departments such as med-surg, ED, and general ICU, nurses who feel rewarded and positively challenged with the wide variety of diagnoses and treatment plans are energized in these settings. They love to learn new things and enjoy ever-changing patient-care areas. If your personality assessment reflects these traits, you may want to seriously consider working there. If your assessment showed that you love learning new things and adapt well to sudden changes around you, then you would probably enjoy this environment.

If you prefer to dive a little deeper into a specialty and are not as interested in constantly switching it up, departments such as specialized ICUs, L&D, or behavioral health might be just the thing for you. In these areas, there is plenty of opportunity to learn new things coupled with a high degree of predictability. Nurses who thrive in these units love getting to know their patient population inside and out. They find joy in going deep, not wide. This allows them to become the go-to expert for a specific kind of care.

These nurses like variety but also appreciate a level of structure. They don't mind seeing similar cases because it allows them to build confidence and expertise. If you're analytical, enjoy problem-solving in a structured way, and prefer some predictability, specialized ICUs (e.g., neuro or burn), behavioral health, or L&D might be a great fit. My assessments revealed that these are dominant traits for me, which makes complete sense. I loved the high stakes of critical care and the mastery I gained for all things related to patients with skin injuries in the burn ICU. There was just enough variety to keep things interesting but not so much that it got in the way of becoming an expert.

CHAPTER 9

Like You, Every Hospital Has Its Own Personality

We've spent a good bit of time exploring what type of units may be a good fit for you, but let's hit pause and zoom out with a wider lens to consider that there are many different types of hospitals as well. The hospital itself—the building you walk into, the system you operate in, the culture you breathe in every single shift—matters just as much as the role you choose.

And yes, I know that "culture" is a buzzword right now. It's slapped on every job posting like an old bumper sticker: *"Supportive team! Collaborative culture! We're like family!"* But here's the truth: culture is more than free pizza and a ping-pong table in the breakroom. It's how you're treated when you make a mistake. It's whether you feel safe speaking up. It's how leadership shows up—or doesn't.

Let me tell you something that would've saved me years of burnout, self-doubt, and 2:00 a.m. "just browsing" job searches like I was on Tinder for trauma centers: the hospital you choose matters.

Not every facility deserves you. Not every system is set up for you to thrive.

> *Culture is more than free pizza and a ping-pong table in the breakroom. It's how you're treated when you make a mistake. It's whether you feel safe speaking up. It's how leadership shows up—or doesn't.*

And if you're an experienced nurse who thinks they hate nursing? You probably don't. You just hate the way your hospital does nursing.

Let's talk about it. All of it. Not just trauma levels and nurse-to-patient ratios but also the environment, the vibe, the people, the paperwork, the politics, and the peace. This chapter breaks down the different types of hospitals you might encounter, from big academic medical centers to tiny rural facilities, and what it's really like to work in each. We also cover the hidden clues you can spot before you ever accept an offer.

After all, this book isn't just about jobs. It's about fit. And you deserve a fit that feels good.

Skylar's Story

I was well into my nursing program, a junior in the accelerated program, with two young kids at home and a husband trying to hold it down while I chased this wild and holy calling. My plate wasn't just full. It was dripping over the sides. But I was determined. I knew I had something to give, even if I didn't know exactly where I fit yet.

I landed my first nurse extern position at a community hospital ICU. On paper, it was a dream. Critical care. High acuity. A chance to dig into the real stuff. I was excited and ready to prove myself. That hospital took a chance on me with zero experience, and I'll always be grateful for that. They opened the door. But here's the part they don't tell you in school: just because you're invited in doesn't mean it's home.

From day one, something felt...off. Not terrible. Not toxic. Just off.

The unit functioned. The nurses were competent. The work got done. But I couldn't shake the feeling that I was constantly trying to shrink myself to fit in. I didn't look forward to my shifts. I didn't feel the buzz of curiosity or connection that I had anticipated experiencing in the ICU. I chalked it up to being

Like You, Every Hospital Has Its Own Personality

new. To imposter syndrome. To being tired from juggling babies and textbooks.

But no matter how I tried to explain it away, the truth was plain: I didn't belong there. And it had nothing to do with my skills or the department I was in.

About a month into it, I got an offer to extern at another hospital's ICU. Bigger hospital. Academic center. More chaos, more variety. I almost didn't apply because I didn't want to seem ungrateful. Did I really need another spot? Wasn't I lucky? Shouldn't I just make it work?

But something in me whispered, "What can it hurt? Just go check it out. You owe it to yourself." So I interviewed and got the offer! From the first shift at that second hospital, it felt different. I walked onto the unit and people made eye contact. Nurses introduced themselves without being prompted. I watched them talk to each other with a kind of ease and respect that didn't feel performative.

The preceptor they paired me with was warm, direct, and absolutely brilliant. She didn't just tell me what to do; she explained the why behind every move. She asked me questions that stretched me—not to test me but to help me grow. I left that shift energized, not drained.

It didn't feel like work most days. I looked forward to it. I craved it. Not because it was easy. It was far from easy. That unit moved fast, the patients were sick, and the team expected a lot. But I could breathe. I could ask questions. I could be myself and still be seen as capable. That kind of safety is rare. And precious.

I tried to do both externships for a while. I really did. I didn't want to burn a bridge. The first hospital had given me a chance, and part of me felt like I owed them something. Plus, I was still fighting that little voice that said, "Don't be a quitter. Maybe it's you."

But life has a way of forcing clarity.

Between 12-hour shifts, classes, clinicals, and bedtime stories with my babies, something had to give. I was on the brink of burning out before I'd even gotten my license. So I made a decision that changed my life.

I let go of the first job.

And I have never regretted it.

The type of unit didn't matter nearly as much as the type of environment.

I worked in the ICU at both hospitals. Same job title. Similar patients. Tubes, vents, drips—all of it. But the feeling of being a nurse in those two places? Worlds apart.

One felt like walking on eggshells. The other felt like stepping into purpose.

But here's the thing: it wasn't that one hospital was better than the other. They were simply different. One was just better for me.

Had I not said yes to that second externship, I might have thought the first one was just how it had to be. That maybe nursing was always going to feel heavy, lonely, transactional.

That clarity changed everything.

It shaped how I chose my first job out of school. It taught me to ask better questions in interviews. It gave me a taste of what's possible when nurses are supported, not just scheduled.

That second hospital became my launching pad. I stayed there as a new grad. I grew roots there. I became a charge nurse, a preceptor, a leader. I built confidence and community and clarity that I still carry with me today. Not because it was perfect. But because it fit.

What started as a hard decision ended up shaping an entire career.

And it all began with a simple truth: The hospital matters. The people matter. The culture matters.

That difference was everything.

The Hospital's Personality

Location, Commute, and the Invisible Tax

I know it sounds basic, but let's start with geography. Where your hospital is located and how far it is from your life will shape your experience more than you think. Is it 15 minutes away or 90? Are you crossing bridges, paying for parking, or fighting downtown traffic just to get to work?

We're talking about far more than gas and tolls here. Think about all the intangibles:

- That commute? That's emotional labor. That's unpaid overtime. That's the hour you could have been sleeping, stretching, or sitting down to a real meal.
- And if you're a new nurse? Adding a grueling commute on top of a steep learning curve can tip you from tired to tapped out.
- Proximity also affects your availability for extra shifts, your safety during night shifts, and your ability to respond to last-minute calls.

> **POWER PLAY:** Map it out. Actually drive your commute before you sign. Do it at the time of day you'd be heading in. See how it feels. The job might be amazing, but if the drive drains you, it's not sustainable. Let's be honest. It may take you an hour to get to the hospital of your dreams, but if you decide that it's worth it, use that commute to level up your reading on Audible or catch up on your favorite podcast. I worked with a nurse who considered herself a "super commuter" and drove two hours from Alabama to the hospital she had been working in for over 10 years. It's whatever works for you!

Academic vs. General Community

Ever feel like you're doing a group project...at work...every day? Welcome to teaching hospitals. They're fast-paced, collaborative, and full of learners. Think med students, interns, residents, and fellows, all rotating, all growing, all asking questions—hopefully.

That can be beautiful. You'll be surrounded by people pushing the envelope, innovating, and trying new things. You'll see rare cases, cutting-edge procedures, and cross-disciplinary teamwork in action. I personally enjoyed having easy access to a provider at some level when I needed that pain med ordered ASAP.

But let's be real. You'll also be giving reports five times, repeating your name to every new white coat, and managing orders that change faster than a TikTok trend.

If you like a challenge, teaching hospitals will stretch you in the best way. But if you crave predictability and autonomy, you may find the constant motion exhausting.

Non-teaching hospitals, on the other hand, tend to be quieter. Fewer interruptions. More direct communication. You'll likely work with seasoned providers who know their patients and place clean, consistent orders. There are fewer residents (a.k.a. "providers under construction"), which can help nurses create routine workflows while partnering with a smaller group of providers where the nurses know what orders to expect and how they work.

That means more space to find your rhythm, build your confidence, and *be* the nurse you trained to be.

There's no right answer here. Just different flavors. One is a concert with 50 musicians tuning up at once. The other is an intimate quartet with your playlist on repeat.

Which one helps *you* shine?

Magnet vs. Non-Magnet: Glitter or Gold?

Magnet status is awarded by the American Nurses Credentialing Center (ANCC), and it's meant to recognize hospitals that create strong nursing environments. These are places where nurses have a voice, professional development is prioritized, and outcomes are solid. It's a big deal in the world of hospital accolades.

But watch out: just because a hospital has Magnet status doesn't mean it's living those values every day.

I've worked with Magnet hospitals where nurses were deeply respected, supported, and involved in decisions that mattered. You could feel it in the staffing, in the collaboration, in the way new nurses were trained and nurtured.

And I've seen amazing nursing cultures in places that didn't have the Magnet designation. Keep in mind that strong leadership, healthy work environments, and nurse-driven change don't always wait for an accreditation.

Magnet can absolutely be a green flag. But it's kind of like a highly rated restaurant—just because it looks good on paper doesn't mean you're going to love the food. Think about it like this: Nobu is a five-star Japanese restaurant that serves some of the best sushi in the country. But what if you're like me and have no desire to eat sushi? I don't care if it's Michelin rated. That yellowtail jalapeño sashimi is not getting anywhere near my mouth!

It comes down to whether the culture matches what you're looking for. You're not just job hunting. You're not chasing prestige or plaques. You're building a career that's sustainable, aligned with your values, and rooted in real support.

And *that* is always more important than a plaque on the hospital wall.

> *Magnet can absolutely be a green flag. But it's kind of like a highly rated restaurant—just because it looks good on paper doesn't mean you're going to love the food.*

Specialty Hospitals: The Hidden Gems

Let's talk about the underdogs of the hospital world, those specialty settings that don't get enough love in nursing school but can absolutely change your life:

1. Oncology Facilities
   This is sacred work. You'll walk with people through the hardest seasons of their lives. You'll learn clinical depth, emotional intelligence, and what it means to *hold space* for someone. It's intense. It's heavy. But it's also some of the most meaningful nursing you'll ever do. These are great places to work as well if you know you want to specialize in oncology.

2. Psychiatric / Mental-Health Facilities
   Psych nurses are warriors of emotional safety. You'll master therapeutic communication, de-escalation, and trauma-informed care. It's not about passing meds. It's about seeing people. Really seeing them. And helping them stabilize, grow, and find their footing. Psych nursing requires boundaries, empathy, and patience. But if mental health matters to you, this work will feed your soul. Want to be a mental-health nurse practitioner? Working in these settings is a great way to gain the clinical acumen and experience that will help you get into the master's program you want.

3. Rehabilitation Hospitals
   Recovery is its own kind of magic. In rehab settings, you'll help people *rebuild* after strokes, injuries, and surgeries. You'll cheer every milestone, from first steps to full independence. These hospitals often have better staffing, slower pace, and deep relationships. It's less adrenaline, more connection. Less chaos, more consistency.

4. Long-Term Acute Care
   LTAC is where you see complex, medically fragile patients who need ICU-level care for weeks, not just days. It's slower paced than critical care but still high stakes, and you'll get to really *know* your patients in a way that most acute-care nurses never do.

5. Hospice
   Hospice nursing is heart-centered work. You'll be managing comfort, supporting families, and fully present for life's final chapter. It's emotionally intense but also deeply human and wildly meaningful.

6. VA Hospitals
   Working at the VA is its own world. You'll be caring for veterans—resilient, diverse, often underserved people with complex stories. The pros? Federal benefits. Strong job security. A mission that matters. You'll likely have union protections, set pay scales, and a clear path to promotion. The cons? Bureaucracy. Paperwork. Slow-moving systems. And a hiring process that might test your patience. But if you value stability, structure, and service, VA nursing can be a powerful path. Just know that it's not fast paced. But it *is* purposeful.

Union vs. Nonunion: Power, Protection, and Politics

Let's get real about labor. In a union hospital, you're backed by a contract. That means staffing ratios, overtime rules, and protections against arbitrary discipline are written down, not just promised. You have recourse if things go sideways. But unions come with dues, politics, and sometimes red tape. Progress can be slow. Tensions can flare.

Nonunion hospitals may offer more flexibility, quicker pivots, and/or closer relationships with leadership. But without formal protections, you, your license, and your career are more exposed.

Either way, know your rights. Read the policies. Document everything. Ask hard questions. And if you're ever in doubt, phone a friend, call the union rep, or reach out to a nurse mentor who knows the ropes.

Your license, your labor, and your lifestyle are worth protecting.

How to Vet a Hospital Before You Say Yes

If I can offer you a couple of pieces of advice when it comes to finding the hospital that has the right personality fit for you, before you accept the job, do this:

1. Drive the commute.
2. Ask about nurse-to-patient ratios.
3. Tour the unit.
4. Watch the nurses talk to each other.
5. Ask, "How long do people stay here?"
6. Ask, "What happens when staffing is short?"
7. Find out if there is a solid shared-governance structure. What decisions are nurses authorized to make?
8. Ask, "Do you support continuing education?"

And my personal favorite?

"May I shadow for a few hours before I decide?"

Reading a job post is like reading a dating profile. It's curated. Filtered. Polished. But walking the halls? Feeling the energy?

That's the real story.

Like You, Every Hospital Has Its Own Personality

Interview Guide

https://auspicious-water-67783.myflodesk.com/m0zdbscmcr

You're Not Asking Too Much; You're Asking the Right Questions

Choosing your hospital isn't about being picky. It's about being aligned. You deserve to work in a place that values your voice, respects your time, and invests in your growth.

Whether you end up in a teaching hospital or a trauma center, a psych facility or a VA system, a Magnet beacon or a community gem, make sure it fits. Not just your skills. Your soul.

Nursing is hard enough without trying to bloom out of soil that is choking the life out of you. Find your fit. And don't settle for less.

And if you're wondering *how* you'll know when it's the right fit? That's where your gut comes in. In the next chapter, we talk about tuning into your instincts, spotting red flags before you're knee-deep in regret, and trusting yourself to choose a path that feels right, not just on paper but also in your bones.

CHAPTER 10

Gut Check

There's a moment, right before you accept your first nursing job, when everything feels both terrifying and electric at the same time.

Your palms are sweaty. Your phone's lit up with "Congratulations!" messages. Everyone's asking where you're going. And you're trying to smile through the nausea in your stomach because deep down, you're still asking yourself:

Did I choose the right unit?
Am I really ready?
What if I hate it?

Let me tell you something. Those questions don't mean you're weak or uncertain. They mean you're *aware*. Aware that this decision is important, not permanent, but pivotal all the same.

Consider this chapter as your gut check. It's not just a recap. It's a reckoning. A moment to pause, reflect, and get honest about what you've learned not just about the profession but about yourself. Finding your fit is not about chasing status or picking what's trendy. It's about learning to trust that quiet, scared voice inside you that knows what *feels* right. Let's walk through it.

Brianna's Breakthrough

I wasn't one of those people who always knew what kind of nurse I wanted to be.

To be honest, I was just trying to survive nursing school. I was exhausted, behind on chapter readings, and praying that my final semester would go by fast. I thought that I'd just take whatever job came my way after graduation and figure it out from there.

But one of my classmates mentioned she was working as a nurse extern and that it was helping her figure out what kind of unit she liked. That got my attention. I didn't know what an externship was before that moment, but I investigated it, applied, and somehow got in.

I wanted ICU. That's where I believed I belonged—high acuity, fast pace, all the bells and whistles. Whenever I thought of nursing, that's what I thought of. But when I asked the nurse manager if I could choose my unit, she shook her head no and said, "Just give it a few months. You can always change. That's the beautiful thing about nursing. But trust me. I'm good at my job and at choosing the right unit for my students."

I didn't love that answer, but I went with it. I just wanted to get into the hospital and see what nursing really looked like.

Then I saw my unit assignment:

Oncology.

I stared at the paper like it might change if I blinked hard enough. I hadn't had a single clinical rotation in oncology. We barely covered it in class. All I knew was that it was emotionally intense and full of very sick patients. I had that sinking feeling in my stomach like maybe this was going to be too much emotionally.

But I kept thinking about what that manager had said. So I didn't push back. I showed up, despite my fear.

I was nervous on my first day. The kind of nervous where your hands are clammy and your voice feels stuck in your throat.

The nurse I was paired with, Patrice, had this quiet presence about her. She didn't need to talk much. You could tell that she knew her stuff just by the way she moved. "You're with me today," she said. That was it. No big intro. Just go time.

We walked into a room where a young woman named Maya was lying in bed. Her head was covered with a soft, faded beanie. She looked pale, weak, and tired.

But she smiled.

"Hi," she uttered, her voice barely above a whisper. "You must be new."

I nodded. I didn't know what to say. Honestly, I didn't feel like I belonged there at all.

I helped with her meds. Held the emesis basin when the nausea kicked in. Adjusted her pillows. Watched as Patrice calmly navigated every beep, every concern, every emotion like it was second nature.

When her daughter showed up to visit, Maya looked at me and said, "Can you help me sit up? I want her to see me looking strong."

That did something to me. Shifted something I didn't have words for yet.

And it was just the beginning.

The days on that unit were long. And some were hard in a way that I wasn't prepared for. I saw families pacing the hall, just trying to hold it together for each other. I saw patients go through unthinkable pain with so much grace it cracked me open.

But it wasn't all heavy.

I saw so much joy too. Real joy. Nurses bringing in balloons for chemo bell days (those are the last days a patient is receiving inpatient chemotherapy and soon to be headed home). Patients making jokes with their doctors like they were old friends. Nursing assistants praying with families before shift change. Laughter, even in the middle of heartbreak.

It was human. All of it.

One day, a patient grabbed my hand after I'd helped her back into bed and said, "You've got a soft heart. Don't lose that."

I hadn't even realized how much I needed to hear those words until she said them.

Now, over two decades later, oncology is still where I feel most like myself.

That externship didn't just give me experience. It gave me clarity. It held up a mirror and showed me who I was before I had the letters behind my name.

If I'd bailed on that unit or waited around for what I thought was the "perfect" placement, I probably would've ended up in a unit that looked good on paper but didn't fit my soul.

Instead, I landed somewhere that taught me how to hold space. How to stay soft in hard moments. How to show up fully without falling apart.

Oncology did that for me.

Turns out that nurse manager was good at her job after all.

You've Been Gathering Receipts

Through these pages so far, we've walked through some of the most common (and chaotic) units in the hospital. You've stood in the noise of the emergency department, where adrenaline feels like currency and the pace can either light you up or burn you out. You've tiptoed through the sacred stillness of oncology, where emotions run deep, and every moment with a patient feels like a shared heartbeat. You've clocked the layered choreography of the ICU, the multitasking madness of med-surg, and the unpredictable miracle zone that is L&D. And each unit taught you something not just about what they require but also about what you need to thrive.

This is like building your own personal nursing compass. Every chapter is another direction. Another clue. Another layer. Let's pull all those threads together and see what your map is really telling you.

Take Inventory: What Have You Learned About *Yourself*?

Before you move forward, stop for a moment and look back. It's time for some introspection.

Ask yourself:

- "What kind of pace makes me feel energized, not drained?"
- "How much emotional weight can I carry before it starts costing me my joy?"
- "Do I thrive on variety and chaos, or do I prefer rhythm and routine?"
- "How important is flexibility and work-life balance for this season of my life?"
- "Do I love independence, or do I need clear direction and strong team collaboration?"
- "How comfortable am I in tech-heavy environments?"
- "Do I want to feel deeply connected to my patients or more task oriented in my day-to-day?"

This is not about picking the "perfect" answers. It's about collecting *honest* ones.

Let me be clear. You're not choosing a forever marriage. You're choosing your next move. One that makes sense for who you are *right now*. That may change; it may not. Either way is okay. That's why you must think about the here and now and not just 5 or 10 years in the future. However, it is a good idea to keep your long-term career goals in the back of your mind.

Let Your Future Guide Your Present

Let's get even more real.

Where do you want this career to take you?

Leadership? Education? Community health? Becoming an NP or CRNA? Diving into public health or research?

Those answers matter because some units will stretch you toward those goals and others will keep you stuck in survival mode.

Let me say this loud for the people in the back: IT'S OKAY IF YOU DON'T KNOW IT YET. You're allowed to be unsure.

You're allowed to have a plan and change it. You're allowed to pivot, redirect, or completely reroute your nursing journey as many times as you need.

That's why matching your unit to your personality is so powerful. Even if you don't have your whole career mapped out, starting in a place that aligns with how you're wired gives you space to breathe, grow, and see clearly what your next step might be.

When you're not constantly battling burnout, imposter syndrome, or chaos that doesn't fit your spirit, you finally have room to explore what you really want.

Your current choice is a stepping stone. Let your future goals inform your direction, but don't let them cage you in.

The most important thing right now is to start where you shine—and trust that clarity will meet you as you move.

But also, don't forget about the culture. Culture is sticky. And no matter how amazing the orientation packet is, if the vibe is off, it won't work. You cannot fully know a unit just from a job posting or a recruiter's pitch. You must experience it. Because remember: units don't change nearly as often as leaders do.

> **POWER PLAY:** Scout the culture. If you can, shadow a nurse in the department. Ask to volunteer. Get an externship or work as a tech before graduation. The earlier you get your eyes and feet in the space, the more clarity you'll have.
> During interviews, ask questions that give you perspective:
> - How does your team support new grads?
> - What happens when a nurse is having a hard shift?
> - How does leadership respond to burnout?
> - How long has the manager been there?
> - How do you handle conflicts and/or communication breakdowns?
>
> And my personal favorite: what's one thing people on this unit love, and what do they wish were different?

Gut Check: No One Knows Better Than You Do

At the end of the day, I want you to really listen to what your mind, body, and spirit are trying to tell you. Not the other nurses, not the patients, not your professors.

When you walk onto a unit, what does your *gut* say?

Are your shoulders tense? Is your chest tight? Or do you feel curious, maybe even excited?

These are all signals your gut is giving you. It's wisdom. It's your nervous system trying to keep you safe and aligned.

And you can 100 percent trust it. Even if other people don't get it. Even if your nursing school bestie is obsessed with the ICU and you're drawn to behavioral health. Even if your professors are pushing you toward "more impressive" units. *Even if your family doesn't understand your decision.*

This is *your* life. *Your* license. *Your* calling.

You don't have to explain your alignment to anyone who isn't walking in your scrubs.

You Belong There

Let me say it plainly: you don't need a perfect résumé, a list of certifications, or a 10-year plan to earn your place in the nursing profession. You belong there because you care.

You belong there because you've done the work to understand who you are and how you want to show up.

You belong there because this book was never about putting you into a mold. It is about giving you permission to shape your own path.

If your gut is telling you something, listen.

If a unit feels wrong in your gut, believe it. You don't need rhyme or reason. You don't even need logic.

If a door opens and it aligns with your energy, trust your gut and walk through it with your head high. That quiet inner voice? It's there for a reason. There's no universal "right" choice, only what feels right for *you*. When you start tuning into that instinct, honoring what lights you up instead of what simply checks a box, you stop chasing someone else's version of success. And that, my friend, is how you build a career that doesn't just pay the bills but also fills your soul.

CHAPTER 11

Go All In

You've made the leap. You've chosen your next space. Be it your first role fresh out of school, a new hospital across town, or a whole new specialty that's been calling your name. You asked the hard questions during the interview. You trusted your gut. You said yes. And now, here you are at the edge of something brand new. Congratulations!

Badge clipped on. Scrubs still stiff from the first wash. That mix of nerves and excitement buzzing under your skin like a second heartbeat. You're officially starting your next chapter.

This is the part nobody prepares you for—not really. Because choosing your next move is only half the battle. What matters now is how you show up in the space you chose. How you plant yourself in new ground and decide, day after day, to grow into the nurse you're meant to be.

And let's be honest. Starting over, even when it's the right choice, can shake you in ways you don't expect. You might miss your old coworkers. You might second-guess yourself when the charting system looks different or the patient flow moves at a speed you're not used to. You might wonder if you made the right call at all. Change can be scary in any situation.

But that fear and doubt you may be feeling is not a sign that you're not ready. It's a sign that you're human. And it's a sign that you're exactly where you're supposed to be.

This chapter is about what happens after the acceptance letter, after the "Welcome to the team!" email. It's about after the first-day jitters wear off and real life kicks in. It's about how to go all in on yourself—how to learn, lead, build your squad, take feedback like a champion, and root yourself deep enough that no storm can shake you loose.

You don't have to be perfect. You just need to be willing. Let's get to work!

Carlos's Chronicle: The Hard Lesson About Feedback

I had swagger. The kind you earn when you make it through nursing school with clinical instructors singing your praises. The kind you wear like armor when you're the first in your family to graduate college. The kind that makes you think that you're ready for anything. I stepped onto the cardiac step-down unit like it was a stage built just for me. My handwritten nursing "brain" in hand, stethoscope around my neck, ready to run the show.

At first, it went exactly how I had pictured. I was able to start IVs on the first stick. Patients loved me! "You remind me of my grandson!" they'd say.

I was the first to jump up when a bed alarm went off. By the end of week two, even some of the crusty charge nurses were giving me nods of approval. And let me tell you, I soaked it in.

When my preceptors pulled me aside to offer tiny nudges—"Carlos, watch your timing on your 6 p.m. meds," "Carlos, make sure you chart your education conversations in real time"—I smiled, nodded, and filed it away under "not urgent." In my mind, urgency meant codes. Urgency meant crashes. Not some nitpicky little documentation reminder.

About six months in, I was off orientation and taking my own assignments. I was handling every shift like an expert and spending most days patting myself on the back for all my progress.

Then I got assigned a heavy load on a stormy Tuesday night. I will never forget. It smelled like wet scrubs and burned coffee. We were short-staffed because of the thunderstorms and flash floods across the state, and I had four patients, including two fresh post-caths and one confused elderly woman trying to climb out of bed every five minutes.

It was chaos. But I had seen worse and figured I could handle it. Besides, the charge nurse would not have given me this assignment if she hadn't thought I could manage, right? "I've got this," I reassured myself.

Around 7:45 p.m., I started my evening rounds. Room 520 was a 62-year-old post-op named Mr. Jenkins—stern, stoic, the kind of guy who would say "I'm fine" even if his leg were falling off. His vitals looked okay at first glance. BP was a little low, but nothing wild. Heart rate a little fast, but Mr. Jenkins had been anxious all day. I brushed it off, making a mental note to recheck after meds.

But I didn't recheck. Not because I didn't care but because, within the next five minutes, three bed alarms blared like a siren symphony down the hall. Another nurse needed help transferring a bariatric patient, the unit secretary was out, and the phone was ringing off the hook. I sprinted through the next hour like someone dodging the sheets of rain that were pouring outside the hospital at that very moment.

At 9:00 p.m., Miss Janie, another nurse with far more experience, strolled in after agreeing to come in and help. She had been a nurse longer than I'd been alive and had a sixth sense about her patients, a kind of invisible radar that beeped whenever something was off. She stopped outside 520. Didn't even touch the chart. Just looked at Mr. Jenkins from the doorway.

"Something ain't right with Mr. Jenkins, Carlos," she said under her breath.

She marched in and checked his pulse manually: hard, fast, thready. She snapped the vitals machine back on. BP was tanking. Heart rate was racing. Sweat was beading on Mr. Jenkins's forehead.

By the time I came running over, the rapid response was already being called.

Standing there in the fluorescent light, heart hammering, I felt the truth sink into my bones: I had missed it. Missed the slow slide. Missed the warning signs. Missed the tiny, almost whisper changes that should have been screaming at me.

And here was the worst part. If Miss Janie hadn't caught it, Mr. Jenkins could've coded, lying right there in that narrow hospital bed, hooked up to machines that beeped politely as his body tried to crash.

I stood frozen while the rapid response team flooded the room. The respiratory therapist was adjusting the oxygen. The charge nurse is starting a second IV line. The resident is barking out orders.

Miss Janie grabbed my arm—not roughly, not angrily, but firmly. It appears she had a sixth sense about her coworkers too. She led me into the med room, closed the door behind us, and leaned against the counter.

"Carlos, you're not bad at this, baby," she said, voice steady.

"But you are green. And you don't know what you don't know yet. That's why feedback ain't optional. It's survival."

I swallowed the lump rising in my throat.

Miss Janie didn't lecture me. She didn't shame me. She taught me with the kind of raw tenderness that only comes from knowing exactly how high the stakes are.

She pulled up the chart, walked me through the vitals trends, and pointed out how Mr. Jenkins's numbers had been whispering for an hour before they started screaming. She showed me what I should have seen. Showed me what I could catch next time.

And for the first time since I'd started, I really listened.

I sat in my car for over an hour after my shift. Rain drumming against the windshield. Scrubs damp with sweat and regret. Replay after replay running through my head.

I had found out later that the charge nurse from the day shift was new at the role and still learning. She didn't anticipate the callouts; she didn't realize that I was just off orientation.

And as a novice, I wasn't experienced enough to know that

I didn't know enough. After months of successfully handling everything that was thrown at me, I was not prepared for the challenge of this shift. I thought about how easy it would be to blame the chaos, the short staffing, the broken system...but deep down, I knew:

The system was broken, yes.

The chaos was real, yes.

But so was my responsibility.

And so was my potential.

Right there under the dim parking-lot lights, I decided that I wouldn't just survive nursing...I would master it. Piece by piece. Mistake by mistake. Lesson by brutal lesson.

I changed after that night. I chased feedback. I asked for mid-shift check-ins. I debriefed after codes, after falls, after near misses, hungry for every scrap of wisdom the seasoned nurses would throw at me. I learned to catch the whispers before they became screams.

And eventually, new grads started coming to me, wide-eyed and terrified, and I would tell them the story of Mr. Jenkins. Tell them about the lesson I learned in a tiny med room from a nurse who could've shamed me but chose not to. I would tell them that feedback isn't failure. It's your life raft in the middle of the storm.

Today, even as a unit director, I still recognize that I will always be learning and that, in nursing, the most dangerous thing you can be isn't inexperienced. It's being unteachable.

Become a Lifelong Learner

While you're building your clinical skills and finding your people, make it your mission to learn from everybody—and I mean *everybody*. Nurses, techs, physicians, housekeeping, dietary. The tech who's been there 15 years can teach you tricks about lifting and patient flow that your nursing-school textbooks never even hinted at. The housekeeper knows which patient rooms have the tricky bed alarms. The cafeteria worker will sometimes spot when a patient is acting a little "off" before anyone else does. Every single person you work with holds a piece of the bigger puzzle. If you're humble enough to notice, you'll become the kind of nurse that people will trust before you even open your mouth.

You never know when a passing comment from a tech about a patient's behavior will tip you off to a critical change. Or when a physician will drop a nugget of wisdom about patient management that sticks with you forever. Every interaction is a chance to level up—as long as you're paying attention.

Find Your Mentor

Once you're in, the next thing you need is a mentor. Notice I didn't say "preceptor" or "manager." Those roles are important too, but they are not the same as a mentor. A preceptor is responsible for making sure you learn the technical and safety aspects of your role. They are your teacher and your evaluator. A manager, or leader, is tasked with staffing, budgets, and organizational goals. They support you, but their primary focus is running the department.

A mentor, however, is someone who commits to walking with you through your development—someone who cheers your wins and helps you navigate your missteps without judgment. They may not even be formally assigned to you. Often, the best mentors are the ones you build relationships with naturally.

Finding a mentor is important because they help you see beyond the immediate chaos of a rough shift. They remind you that growth is messy. They normalize the fears you think you're not supposed to have. If you don't find a mentor right away, don't panic. Watch for the nurses who are generous with their time, who correct you with kindness, and who take pride in helping others grow. Those are the ones who can become your lifeline.

Accept Constructive Feedback

Another critical piece of going all in is learning how to accept constructive feedback. I know—it's not easy. No one likes being told that they missed something or need to improve, especially when you're already feeling the heavy weight of "Am I good enough?" on your shoulders. But let me say this clearly: feedback is not an attack. It's a gift.

No matter how much you think you know, you will never know everything. Healthcare is always changing. There will always be new best practices, new technologies, and new patient-care strategies. Staying open to learning isn't just a good career move. It's a patient-safety issue.

Every nurse, no matter how experienced, started out unsure and rough around the edges. Dr. Patricia Benner's work with the Dreyfus Model of Skills Acquisition reminds us that expertise isn't born. It's built.

We all begin as novices, gradually progressing to advanced beginner, competent, proficient, and finally expert—not through perfection but through real-world practice, critical reflection, and, yes, feedback.

Constructive criticism is one of the ways we grow from stage to stage. It's not about being *shamed* into change; it's about being *shaped* into the kind of nurse who thinks faster, acts sharper, and cares more deeply because you allowed yourself to learn from every experience, even the uncomfortable ones.

How to Handle Tough Feedback

When you receive constructive criticism, the first thing to do is breathe. Not the shallow, panicked kind—the real kind. In through your nose, out through your mouth, like you're about to enter a patient's isolation room and need to get your game face on.

Then listen. Really listen. Assume that the person giving it to you wants you to succeed unless they flat-out prove otherwise. Most of the time, experienced nurses aren't trying to tear you down but rather they're trying to keep you—and your patients—safe.

If the feedback stings—and it will sometimes—give yourself space to feel it, but don't let it build walls around your heart. Write it down. Sit with it. Ask yourself, "Is there even a tiny bit of truth in this?"

- If the answer is yes, take that piece and grow from it.
- If the answer is truly no, and you've double-checked your ego at the door, just let it go, like a bad pop song.

Either way, you win because you're staying open to becoming better.

Why Showing Up Matters

Unit activities matter more than you think. When you show up to the potluck, the holiday decorating contest, the "crazy sock" day, you're doing more than just making memories. You're building trust. You're weaving yourself into the fabric of a community that will either hold you up or let you fall. And it starts with showing up.

Build Your Squad

Once you get involved, you'll find your squad—and your squad is everything. These are the people who will swap shifts with you when your kid wakes up puking at 3:00 a.m. The ones who will watch your patients during your break without making you feel guilty. The ones who will catch you when you're spiraling after a rough code and remind you that you're not alone.

Building your squad isn't about cliques or popularity contests. It's about identifying the nurses and staff who are invested in the team, not just themselves. It's the nurse who smiles and asks if you need help when you're drowning. It's the tech who high-fives you when you finally get that stubborn IV in. It's the charge nurse who pulls you aside and says, "You're doing better than you think."

Find your people. Nurture those relationships. Protect them.

Invest in More Than Just Your Shift

I get it—you're tired. You're working 12-hour shifts that somehow turn into 15-hour marathons. You want to clock out, go home, and not think about anything healthcare related until your next shift. And you absolutely need your rest (protect it with your life!). But here's the secret sauce that most people don't tell you about: the real opportunities, the ones that plant seeds for your future, often happen outside your assigned shift.

Volunteering to be on a shared-governance council. Agreeing to take on the role of safety champion. Offering to help with a unit project. Though these things are unpaid in the moment, they're actually investments in yourself. They're planting seeds in a garden you're going to want to harvest in a year or two when you're thinking about promotions, specialties, or grad school.

It doesn't have to be all at once. You don't have to be the "yes" person for everything. Maintain boundaries and pick one thing. Dip your toe in. Get visible in ways that matter—not by being the loudest but by being the most consistently engaged. When leadership sees you showing up for the profession and not just the paycheck, they will remember your name when opportunities come knocking.

Your Future Starts Now

Going all in doesn't mean burning yourself out. It means investing smartly. Advocating for yourself from the beginning. Seeking out learning opportunities. Staying humble and hungry. Accepting feedback with grace. And building connections that will turn colleagues into family.

You worked too hard to get here to just survive. You gave up your time, money, and maybe a little dignity along the way. It's time to jump into the deep end and get everything you want out of this career: the fulfillment, the sense of pride, the education, and, ultimately, financial stability!

It's time to thrive.

It's time to go all in.

CHAPTER 12

Your Journey from Self-Doubt to Self-Confidence

Finding your fit isn't a one-time event; it's a lifelong conversation between who you are now and who you are becoming. As you grow, your career should too. This chapter is your permission slip to adapt, evolve, and pivot with power.

Nursing is not a "one and done" career. It's a living, breathing journey, one that grows and stretches with you. Finding your fit isn't just about landing your first job. It's about continuing to check in with yourself, reevaluating where you are, and pivoting when you need to. Life isn't a straight line, and neither is your nursing career. Growth doesn't work that way.

Let's talk about how you stay in tune with your evolution and why that's one of the most important skills you can develop.

Dayna's Diary (That's Me...LOL)

Let me share something straight from my own life. I've lived the pivot more times than I can count. Not because I was lost. Not because I was failing. But because life was calling me to grow, and I chose to listen.

I didn't even start in nursing. My first career was in corporate marketing and advertising—suits, deadlines, strategy meetings, the whole thing. It looked good on paper. But deep down, I knew something was missing. I wanted my work to mean something in a way I could feel in my bones. So I made my first big pivot into nursing.

I traded in power suits for scrubs. Boardrooms for hydrotherapy rooms. And I'll tell you that nothing could've prepared me for how deeply that choice would shape who I was becoming.

I started in trauma and burns—the fire, the adrenaline, the constant intensity. We moved fast and made decisions faster. Shifts often felt like being in a war zone. Some days, the victories were small but sacred: holding a hand, closing a wound, whispering encouragement into the smoke and chaos. That first season taught me resilience like I'd never known before. It taught me how to stand steady when everything around me was on fire. But as life evolved, so did my own needs and wants.

I got injured on the job—a moment that could've been a dead end to my nursing career. Instead, it became a crossroads. My body needed a different pace. And my spirit, if I'm honest,

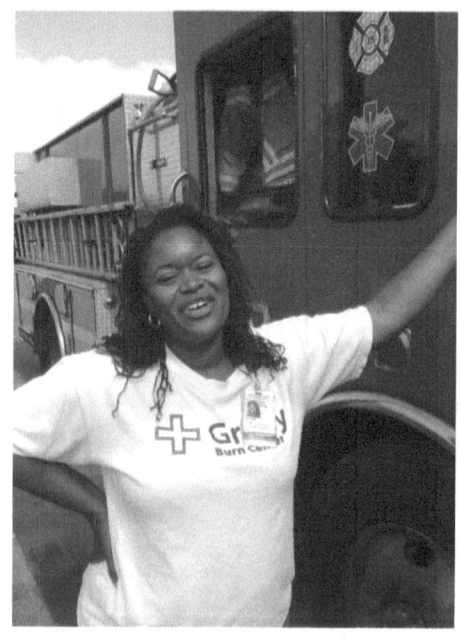

Self-Confidence

was craving something new too. I pivoted again, this time into burns and trauma program management, quality improvement, and education leadership. It was a different kind of intensity. Systems instead of splints. Data dashboards instead of cardiac monitors. I built programs from scratch. I mentored nurses who reminded me so much of myself in those early days. I pushed for change in ways that rippled far beyond any single patient room.

It reminded me of the feeling I had after the first time a patient of mine coded in the ICU and I was able to do CPR and we brought him back. It was terrifying and nerve-wracking but also fulfilling to know that I was able to use my knowledge to have a good outcome in a high-stakes situation.

Next pivot: I moved from burns and trauma leadership into system-wide quality leadership. With it came a bigger playground and a broader impact. I was shaping not just units but entire hospitals. And just when I thought I had found my forever lane with this satisfying work, life nudged me. I got the itch to challenge myself once again.

Once my kids were older and my less hectic home life afforded me a little more breathing room, I leaned back into operational leadership. That meant the 24/7 responsibility of running entire units. Managing crises that didn't wait for business hours. Being the person everyone looked to when the pressure hit its peak. It wasn't easy, but it was a full-circle moment. Every skill, every lesson, every scar I'd picked up along the way came into sharp focus. It made me a stronger leader because I hadn't just read the manuals; I had lived them.

And then came another pivot, this time into executive leadership. I was leading the teams that welcomed me into nursing: the nurse externship and nurse-residency programs. This full-circle moment brought me back to the hospital where my nursing story had first begun. I was walking those halls again, but this time with a different purpose. A bigger voice. A deeper responsibility to the nurses and patients who walked those floors.

What now? Another pivot, perhaps the biggest one yet.

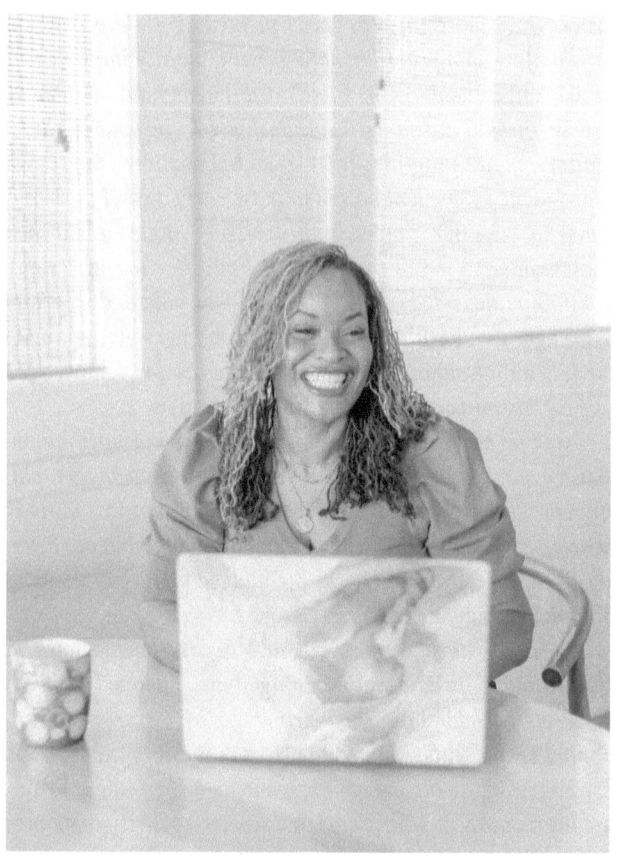

Entrepreneurship. Authorship. Building programs that empower nurses to find their fit. Coaching nurses who are on the edge of burnout or self-doubt or career confusion and helping them step into their power. Writing the words I wish someone had spoken to me when I was doubting myself at 23, or 33, or even yesterday.

Each pivot wasn't about starting over. It was about leveling up. It was about paying attention to what my life was trying to tell me and trusting that even if I couldn't see the full map and a higher power was guiding me in the right direction, all I needed to do was listen to HIM.

Choosing Your Path (and Protecting Your Peace)

Say you decide that you want to work in the ER—that adrenaline, that "anything can happen" energy. Amazing! But if you know that you're someone who needs time to emotionally reset, then part of choosing the ER will also be choosing to fiercely protect your mental health. You might need regular mental-health check-ins, scheduled time off, therapy, or a solid debriefing practice to help you process the high-intensity scenes you'll witness.

Or maybe you're drawn to the ICU. You love the complexity, the challenge, the way one patient can consume your whole brain's focus. That's a beautiful thing. But ICU life also demands a different kind of emotional resilience—one that comes from sitting with the reality that sometimes, despite all our skills, patients don't get better. Choosing ICU means choosing to build those coping skills alongside your technical ones.

Maybe your pull is toward med-surg, a phenomenal place to build strong clinical foundations, but time management has never been your strongest suit. That's not a dealbreaker; it's a skill you can actively work on in a lower-stakes environment before moving into units where the distractions come hard and fast.

The choice of department is never just about where you want to be. It's also about recognizing what you need to support yourself to be your best emotionally, mentally, and physically.

Let Yourself Be Surprised

Here's one of the coolest parts about nursing. You are going to discover talents you didn't even know you had. Maybe you always pictured yourself in the ICU, but after floating to behavioral health, you realize that you have a gift for connecting with patients in crisis. Maybe you thought you wanted the ED forever, but after becoming a preceptor, you realize that your heart is in

> *Stay open to those surprises. Sometimes the very experiences that scare us the most end up showing us who we're meant to become.*

mentoring new nurses. Stay open to those surprises. Sometimes the very experiences that scare us the most end up showing us who we're meant to become.

You may even discover that a skill you once considered a "weakness" turns out to be your greatest strength in a different context. Your ability to stay calm under pressure might shine brighter in the chaos of the ER than it ever did during nursing school simulations. Your love for patient education might bloom fully when you step into a diabetes-management clinic. Nursing holds space for all of it.

Growth Requires Reevaluation

Growth isn't something you feel happening in real time. Growth is something you realize when you pause, breathe, and look around. Make it a habit to reevaluate yourself every year or so. What skills have you built that weren't there before? What's gotten easier for you? What's still a struggle? What's lighting you up, and what's draining you dry?

Maybe, after a couple of years crushing it in med-surg, you're ready to test out your ability to thrive in the ER. Maybe, after spending time in a high-acuity ICU, you realize that you want a different kind of patient connection and decide to try oncology or palliative care.

Or maybe you realize that you want a completely different pace altogether, a pivot toward school nursing, case management, or telehealth.

Reevaluation isn't admitting failure. It's honoring your progress. It's checking your internal compass and making course corrections that align with who you are now and not who you were when you first pinned on that badge.

Pivoting in Nursing...and in Life

Nursing is a career built for pivots, because life will keep shifting—and so will you.

Your path will be uniquely yours. It won't look like mine or anybody else's. And that's exactly how it's supposed to be. But hear me when I say that this pivoting is not a sign of failure. It's a sign that you are still growing. Still answering the call. Still becoming the nurse, the leader, the human you are meant to be.

Keep listening. Keep moving. You're not behind. You're building something bigger than you can even see right now. Trust the pivot, because only then will you see that your abilities are limitless.

When it comes to making a career change, I want you to remember that no test, no assessment, no checklist defines you. Period. The strengths you identified when you first started this journey are important, and they give you a foundation to build on. But they are not the ceiling for what you can achieve. They are starting points, not finish lines. And starting points mean that you have a journey ahead of you—a journey filled with detours and potential pivots.

Matching your skills to a unit is guidance, not a prison sentence. It's about understanding where you can thrive right now based on who you are today. But people change. Skills deepen. Life happens. And you deserve the freedom to change right along with it.

Those early assessments help you know what natural gifts you bring to your patients and where you might want to do a little extra prep work. Maybe you're wired for fast-paced environments, or you're a natural relationship builder who thrives in departments that need emotional intelligence front and center. That self-awareness gives you a powerful head start, but it will never be a straight and narrow road.

> *Nursing is a career built for pivots, because life will keep shifting—and so will you.*

Life Changes = Career Changes (and That's Okay)

Life outside work changes too. You fall in love. You get married. You have a baby. You take on caregiving roles in your family. You go back to school. Each life change shifts what you need from your career.

Maybe working three 12-hour night shifts was perfect when you were single and energized by overtime. Maybe it's not sustainable now that you're juggling childcare or building a business. Maybe you loved the physical challenge of med-surg when you were 22, but now you're thinking long term and want a role that's a little less taxing on your knees and back.

Listening to Your Heart

Sometimes your pivot won't come from logistics, skills, or life circumstances. Sometimes it will come from a deep, emotional knowledge that something has shifted inside you.

You might wake up one morning and realize that the unit you once loved now leaves you feeling hollow. You might notice that the joy you used to feel when advocating for your patients has been replaced by exhaustion you can't shake off. You might sit in your car after a shift and realize that you don't recognize yourself anymore.

If that moment comes, listen.

Emotional pivots are just as valid and just as necessary as logistical ones. Sometimes your heart knows that it's time to move on before your mind can even articulate why.

Emotional pivots are just as valid and just as necessary as logistical ones. Sometimes your heart knows that it's time to move on before your mind can even articulate why.

Maybe you once thrived on the adrenaline of trauma cases, but now you crave the steadier rhythm of a specialty clinic.

Maybe you once lived for the chaos of the ED, but now you want to build deeper, longer-term relationships with patients in a different setting.

This doesn't mean you're "burning out" in a way that can only be fixed with time off. It might mean you've outgrown the environment that once fit you perfectly. That, my friend, is evolution; it's growth.

Giving yourself permission to pivot based on emotional needs is one of the most powerful ways to protect your passion for this work long term. Doing so isn't running away. It's running toward a version of nursing and a version of yourself that continues to light you up from the inside out.

Beyond the Bedside

When talking about career growth in nursing, a lot of people automatically think bedside or nurse practitioner. But nursing is so much bigger than that.

You could become any of the following:

- **Nurse educator** teaching the next generation of nurses
- **Infection preventionist** protecting patients and staff from healthcare-associated infections
- **Case manager** helping patients navigate complex discharges and care transitions
- **Quality-improvement specialist** analyzing processes and improving patient outcomes
- **Clinical-research nurse** working on groundbreaking studies that shape future treatments
- **Health-policy advocate** changing the system from the legislative side
- **Telehealth nurse** providing virtual care and reaching patients across geographic barriers

- **Legal nurse consultant** advising on healthcare-related legal cases
- **Entrepreneur** starting your own business, consulting, coaching, writing
- **Insurance nurse consultant** reviewing medical claims and advocating for patients
- **Medical-device specialist** training staff on new technologies and advancing healthcare innovation
- **Pharmaceutical company educator or liaison** bridging clinical practice with medication management and new therapies
- **Healthcare design consultant** working with architectural firms to design more functional, patient-centered hospitals and clinics

The opportunities are endless. The beauty is that you don't have to have your whole path mapped out today. But you must stay open, curious, and willing to step into the next version of yourself when the time comes.

Progress over Perfection

Listen, no one gets this journey "perfect." Not me. Not the nurse with 20 years' experience. Not the new grad who seems to have it all figured out. What is "perfect" anyway?

Nursing, just like life, is about progress over perfection. It's about making the best decisions you can with the information you have today and giving yourself permission to update those decisions when your information—or your needs—change.

Every pivot, every shift, every reevaluation is a sign of wisdom, not weakness. It means you're paying attention. It means you're honoring your growth.

Stay open. Stay curious. Stay willing to change.

You're not just building a career.
You're building a life.

The Nurse You Are Becoming

When you first opened this book, you may have been feeling overwhelmed. Maybe you were wondering if you would ever find your place in this vast, demanding world of nursing. Maybe you were still standing on what we call the "Island of Anxiety," looking across the water and hoping and praying that the "Land of Confidence" was real.

Now, after walking through these pages together, I hope you can see that it is very real.

You didn't just read about unit vibes or work-life balance or emotional energy...you *felt* the truth in those lessons. You didn't just take inventory of your strengths...you *claimed* them. You didn't just explore different specialties...you *gave yourself permission* to choose the one that fits who you are, not who they think you're supposed to be.

You didn't just read the stories shared by nurses across a wide variety of specialties from across the country...you shared their lived experiences.

At the beginning of this journey, I set out to write a book that would help you figure out where you fit. A book that would help you gain insights into how to assess different nursing specialties, align your natural talents with the needs of various departments, and build a career that fuels both your professional growth and personal fulfillment. And here you are.

You have the tools now. You have the insights. Most importantly, you have the deep, lived understanding that finding your fit isn't a one-time event. Finding your fit is a lifelong practice of knowing yourself and honoring that knowledge with bold, courageous action.

> *You've taken the time to know yourself. You are brave enough to seek alignment, not approval. You understand that your fit is yours to create, again and again, as you grow.*

Finding your fit isn't about chasing perfection. It's about finding alignment between your skills, your spirit, your season of life, and the environment around you. And alignment doesn't happen by accident. It happens because you are brave enough to listen to your own voice over all the noise. It happens because you are wise enough to adapt, evolve, and pivot when the time is right.

This profession will continue to stretch you and change you. Nursing will ask for your hands, your mind, your heart, and sometimes even your soul. But if you keep honoring your growth the way you have throughout this journey, you won't just survive—you'll thrive.

Wherever you go next—whether it's a high-adrenaline trauma unit, a peaceful outpatient clinic, a classroom, a policy boardroom, or a business you build with your own two hands—I hope you never forget:

You are not standing on the Island of Anxiety anymore. You are already walking with confidence, with purpose, and with power into the career and the life you were always meant to build.

You've taken the time to know yourself. You are brave enough to seek alignment, not approval. You understand that your fit is yours to create, again and again, as you grow.

And that, my beautiful friend, is something to be proud of.

Acknowledgments

This book was not written in tidy sessions or compiled in perfect order.

It was written in fragments—over years, between jobs, late at night when the words flowed, during quiet mornings before the world had woken up and life had started "life-ing." It was carried in my chest long before it ever lived on the page.

And if I'm honest, *it almost didn't happen.*

There were times when I questioned whether I had anything left to say and whether the system had already taken too much of my passion. But every time I considered stepping away from the words, I'd hear from another nurse who would remind me why this work matters. A new grad in tears, unsure if she belonged. A seasoned nurse worn down from carrying too much for too long. A nurse leader burned out trying to protect patients, the system, and the team.

It became clear: We weren't the problem. We were the proof.

Like a patient who finally changes his eating habits after the scare of a near-fatal heart attack, it took experiencing the devastating mistreatment from a leader to make me think differently about my frustrations and desires. To make me want to get off the sidelines, speak my truth, and help others stop deferring their dreams and start living their best nursing life!

To God, thank you to my Lord and Savior, Jesus Christ.

To my parents, your steady strength taught me that love is leadership. Your legacy lives in every life I've touched and will touch through this work. Thank you for cultivating a love of books and reading in our home!

To my husband, your unwavering support and belief in my ability to accomplish anything I set my mind to has carried me through the times when I wondered if I would ever get to see this dream become a reality.

To my sister, my ride-or-die. You have always encouraged me and listened to my wins and losses, my ups and downs. *Thank you for being down with me like four flat tires!*

To my son—becoming your mother was the moment I stepped into the most sacred role of my life. You made me "Mom," and that changed everything. Your inquisitive intelligence, relentless work ethic, and sheer kindness make me proud. Thank you for encouraging me not to be intimidated by TikTok!

To my daughter, whose very existence redefined my understanding of purpose. You are the reason I write with truth and walk with integrity. You came into this world living life fearlessly and inspiring me to do the same. I hope that this book is an example of what it looks like when a woman uses her voice, even when it shakes.

To all the nurses who allowed me to share your stories in this book. Your vulnerability and wisdom gave these pages a heartbeat. Without your stories, it is just another tip sheet. Your lived experiences aren't just told here. They helped shape the lens through which this entire book was written. Thank you for letting me bear witness.

To Jessica, who didn't let me off the hook. You said, "Write the damn book," and I did. That push mattered.

To Amelia Forczak, Deanna Novak, and Karen Rowe with Pithy Wordsmithery, thank you for all of your support, expertise, and cheerleading. I am so grateful to you for keeping me on time and honest with this work. Amelia, the day you told me I had the talent to write this, my first book, I was empowered to share my story even more.

To every nurse who has ever felt overwhelmed or helpless, wondered whether they chose the wrong profession, searched for

Acknowledgments

their fit in systems that don't fit everyone, or felt too tender, too tired, too unsure but kept going anyway…

…you are the reason I wrote this book.

This is not just a collection of stories or strategies. It is a hand extended across breakrooms and hospital halls. It is an affirmation that you are not alone in this. And more than that, it is a reminder:

You were never meant to fit into a system that doesn't see your full worth. You were meant to build a career that honors who you are.

Start where you shine. Find your fit.

And if no one's told you lately, you're doing way better than you give yourself credit for!

About the Author

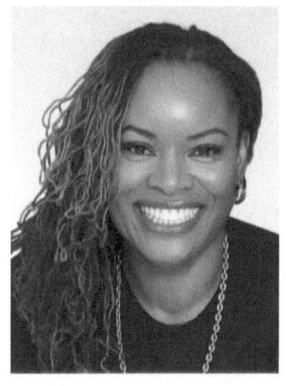

Dr. Dayna Vidal, known as "Dr. Day," is a nationally recognized healthcare executive and thought leader in clinical quality, patient safety, and nursing professional development. She started her medical career as a nurse in the burn ICU after 10 years in corporate marketing and currently serves as patient-safety officer at Wilson Medical Center, a Duke LifePoint hospital, leading system-wide initiatives in quality improvement, regulatory compliance, and organizational safety. With over a decade of leadership experience—much of it dedicated to advancing nursing education, nursing practice, and workforce development—Dr. Vidal has helped shape the careers of countless healthcare professionals through innovative residency models, simulation-based learning, and evidence-based practice frameworks. Her deep expertise in professional development informs her work as a career coach and published author. Dr. Vidal has mentored and coached hundreds of both experienced and new grad nurses through successful career starts and pivots. Triple board-certified, she is a sought-after speaker on high-reliability systems, health equity, career advancement, and leadership. She brings a strategic, people-centered approach to transforming care delivery through education, mentorship, and advocacy.

A native of Atlanta, Georgia, Dayna is married to her college sweetheart, Kwame, and enjoys spending time with her two children, Kimani and Kaylin, and the family fur babies, Honey and Tuko.

Endnotes

i   Lydia Saad, "Americans' Ratings of U.S. Professions Stay Historically Low," *Gallup*, January 13, 2025, https://news.gallup.com/poll/655106/americansratingsprofessionsstayhistoricallylow.aspx.

ii   Heather K.S. Laschinger and Roberta Frida, "New Nurses Burnout and Workplace Wellbeing: The Influence of Authentic Leadership and Psychological Capital," *Science Direct*, April 2, 2014, https://www.sciencedirect.com/science/article/pii/S2213058614000059.

iii   A.O. Bataweel, "Personality Traits, Thinking Styles, and Emotional Intelligence in Nursing, towards Healthcare Providers' Characterization and Safer Patient Care," *Open Journal of Nursing*, 2023, https://www.scirp.org/journal/paperinformation?paperid=123418.

iv   Patricia Benner, *From Novice to Expert: Excellence and Power in Clinical Nursing Practice* (Prentice Hall, 1984).

v   Simon Sinek, *Start with Why: How Great Leaders Inspire Everyone to Take Action* (Portfolio, December 27, 2011).

vi   Almudena Velando-Soriano et al., "Burnout and Personality Factors Among Surgical Area Nurses: A Cross Sectional Multicentre Study," *Frontiers in Public Health*, July 22, 2024, https://pubmed.ncbi.nlm.nih.gov/39104889/.

vii   Chiara Dall'Ora, Jane Ball, Maria Reinius, and Peter Griffiths, "Burnout in nursing: a theoretical review," *Human Resources for Health*, June 5, 2020, https://pubmed.ncbi.nlm.nih.gov/32503559/.

viii   "Qualities of a Great Nurse: A Comprehensive List," HealthStream, April 14, 2021, https://www.healthstream.com/resource/blog/personality-traits-of-a-great-nurse.

ix   Jasmine Vergauwe, Bart Wille, Marjolein Feys, Filip De Fruyt, and Frederik Anseel, "Fear of Being Exposed: The Trait-Relatedness of the Impostor Phenomenon and Its Relevance in the Work Context," *Journal of Business and Psychology*, October 4, 2014, https://doi.org/10.1007/s10869-014-9382-5.

x   Dena M. Bravata et al., "Prevalence, Predictors, and Treatment of Imposter Syndrome: A Systematic Review," *Journal of General Internal Medicine*, December 17, 2019, https://link.springer.com/article/10.1007/s11606-019-05364-1.

xi   Mélanie Lavoie-Tremblay et al., "Nursing Leaders' Perceptions of the Impact of the Strengths-Based Nursing and Healthcare Leadership

xii   Program Three Months Post Training," *International Journal of Nursing Studies Advances*, June 2024, https://doi.org/10.1016/j.ijnsa.2024.100190.

xii   "The Role of Strengths-Based Development in Employee Performance and Engagement," *Gallup Journal of Workplace Research*, https://www.gallup.com.

xiii   "All About the Myers-Briggs® (MBTI®) Assessment," The Myers-Briggs Company, https://www.themyersbriggs.com/en-US/Campaigns/All-About-the-MBTI-Assessment.

xiv   Naeha Pathak, Claire Price, Christina M. Cruz, and Matthew A. Weissman "Using DiSC Personality Tests to Develop Leadership Skills in Internal Medicine Residents," AAPL, May 1, 2025, https://www.physicianleaders.org/articles/doi/10.55834/plj.6712415113.

xv   American Nurses Association, *Nursing: Scope and Standards of Practice*, 3rd Edition (American Nurses Association, 2015).

xvi   D. A. Boyle, "Countering Compassion Fatigue: A Requisite Nursing Agenda," *The Online Journal of Issues in Nursing*, January 31, 2011, https://pubmed.ncbi.nlm.nih.gov/21800933/.

xvii   Christina Maslach and Michael P. Leiter, "Understanding the Burnout Experience: Recent Research and its Implications for Psychiatry," *National Library of Medicine* June 5, 2015, https://pmc.ncbi.nlm.nih.gov/articles/PMC4911781/.

xviii   Christopher C. Imes and Eileen R. Chasens, "Rotating Shifts Negatively Impacts Health and Wellness Among Intensive Care Nurses," *Journal of Nursing Management*, March 2, 2019, https://journals.sagepub.com/doi/10.1177/2165079918820866.

xix   Louise Hall, Judith Johnson, Ian Watt, Anastasia Tsipa, and Daryl B. O'Connor, "Healthcare Staff Wellbeing, Burnout, and Patient Safety: A Systematic Review," *PLOS One*, July 8, 2016, https://journals.plos.org/plosone/article?id=10.1371/journal.pone.0159015&utm_source=plos&utm_medium=email&utm_campaign=PLOS-1705-ALMTOPONE.

xx   NSI Nursing Solutions, *2023 NSI National Health Care Retention & RN Staffing Report*, Workplace Change Collaborative (2023), https://www.wpchange.org/resources/2023-nsi-national-health-care-retention-rn-staffing-report.

xxi   Hilde Myhren, Oivind Ekeberg, and Olav Stokland, "Job Satisfaction and Burnout among Intensive Care Unit Nurses and Physicians," Critical Care Research and Practice, November 5, 2013, https://pubmed.ncbi.nlm.nih.gov/24303211/.

xxii   Rose O. Sherman, EdD, RN, FAAN, "The Myth that Nurses Leave Nursing," *Emerging RN Leader*, November 11, 2013, https://emergingrnleader.com/the-myth-that-nurses-leave-nursing/.

xxiii   "Scope of Practice," American Nurses Association, https://www.nursingworld.org/practice-policy/scope-of-practice/.

www.ingramcontent.com/pod-product-compliance
Lightning Source LLC
Chambersburg PA
CBHW030446100526
44580CB00001B/6

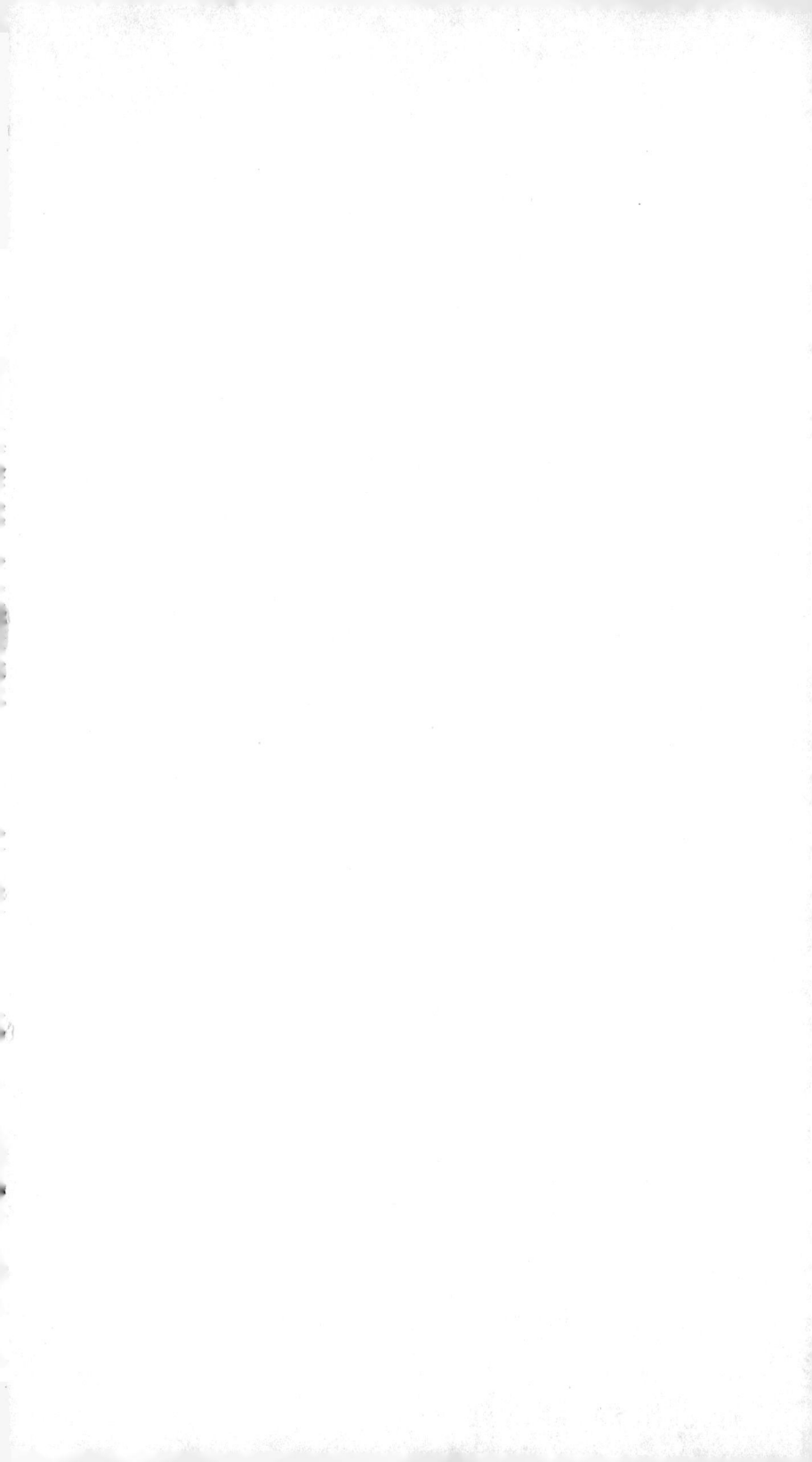